T0358923

Bone Grafts, Bone Graft Substitutes, and Biologics in Foot and Ankle Surgery

Editor

SHELDON S. LIN

FOOT AND ANKLE CLINICS

www.foot.theclinics.com

Consulting Editor
MARK S. MYERSON

December 2016 • Volume 21 • Number 4

ELSEVIER

1600 John F. Kennedy Boulevard • Suite 1800 • Philadelphia, Pennsylvania, 19103-2899

http://www.theclinics.com

FOOT AND ANKLE CLINICS Volume 21, Number 4
December 2016 ISSN 1083-7515, ISBN-13: 978-0-323-47739-0

Editor: Lauren Boyle
Developmental Editor: Meredith Clinton

© 2016 Elsevier Inc. All rights reserved.

This periodical and the individual contributions contained in it are protected under copyright by Elsevier, and the following terms and conditions apply to their use.

Photocopying

Single photocopies of single articles may be made for personal use as allowed by national copyright laws. Permission of the Publisher and payment of a fee is required for all other photocopying, including multiple or systematic copying, copying for advertising or promotional purposes, resale, and all forms of document delivery. Special rates are available for educational institutions that wish to make photocopies for non-profit educational classroom use. For information on how to seek permission visit www.elsevier.com/permissions or call: (+44) 1865 843830 (UK)/(+1) 215 239 3804 (USA).

Derivative Works

Subscribers may reproduce tables of contents or prepare lists of articles including abstracts for internal circulation within their institutions. Permission of the Publisher is required for resale or distribution outside the institution. Permission of the Publisher is required for all other derivative works, including compilations and translations (please consult www.elsevier.com/permissions).

Electronic Storage or Usage

Permission of the Publisher is required to store or use electronically any material contained in this periodical, including any article or part of an article (please consult www.elsevier.com/permissions). Except as outlined above, no part of this publication may be reproduced, stored in a retrieval system or transmitted in any form or by any means, electronic, mechanical, photocopying, recording or otherwise, without prior written permission of the Publisher.

Notice

No responsibility is assumed by the Publisher for any injury and/or damage to persons or property as a matter of products liability, negligence or otherwise, or from any use or operation of any methods, products, instructions or ideas contained in the material herein. Because of rapid advances in the medical sciences, in particular, independent verification of diagnoses and drug dosages should be made.

Although all advertising material is expected to conform to ethical (medical) standards, inclusion in this publication does not constitute a guarantee or endorsement of the quality or value of such product or of the claims made of it by its manufacturer.

Foot and Ankle Clinics (ISSN 1083-7515) is published quarterly by Elsevier, Inc., 360 Park Avenue South, New York, NY 10010-1710. Months of issue are March, June, September, and December. Periodicals postage paid at New York, NY, and additional mailing offices. Subscription price per year is $320.00 (US individuals), $466.00 (US institutions), $100.00 (US students), $360.00 (Canadian individuals), $560.00 (Canadian institutions), $215.00 (Canadian students), $460.00 (international individuals), $560.00 (international institutions), and $215.00 (international students). To receive student/resident rate, orders must be accompanied by name of affiliated institution, date of term, and the *signature* of program/residency coordinator on institution letterhead. Orders will be billed at individual rate until proof of status is received. Foreign air speed delivery is included in all *Clinics* subscription prices. All prices are subject to change without notice. **POSTMASTER:** Send address changes to *Foot and Ankle Clinics*, Elsevier Health Sciences Division, Subscription Customer Service, 3251 Riverport Lane, Maryland Heights, MO 63043. **Customer Service: 1-800-654-2452 (US and Canada). From outside of the United States and Canada, call 314-447-8871. Fax: 314-447-8029. E-mail: JournalsCustomerService-usa@ elsevier.com (for print support); JournalsOnlineSupport-usa@elsevier.com (for online support).**

Reprints. For copies of 100 or more, of articles in this publication, please contact the Commercial Reprints Department, Elsevier Inc., 360 Park Avenue South, New York, NY 10010-1710. Tel.: 212-633-3874; Fax: 212-633-3820; E-mail: reprints@elsevier.com.

Contributors

CONSULTING EDITOR

MARK S. MYERSON, MD
Medical Director, The Foot and Ankle Association, Inc.; Institute for Foot and Ankle Recon at Mercy, Baltimore, Maryland

EDITOR

SHELDON S. LIN, MD
Associate Professor, Department of Orthopaedics, Rutgers New Jersey Medical School, Doctor's Office Center, Newark, New Jersey

AUTHORS

SAMUEL B. ADAMS, MD
Assistant Professor, Department of Orthopaedic Surgery, Duke University Medical Center, Durham, North Carolina

JOHN G. ANDERSON, MD
Orthopaedic Associates of Michigan, Grand Rapids, Michigan

TREENA LIVINGSTON ARINZEH, PhD
Professor, Department of Biomedical Engineering, New Jersey Institute of Technology, Newark, New Jersey

JUDITH F. BAUMHAUER, MD, MPH
Associate Chair of Academic Affairs, Department of Orthopaedics, University of Rochester School of Medicine and Dentistry, Rochester, New York

CHRISTOPHER BIBBO, DO, DPM
Department of Orthopaedics, The Rubin Institute for Advanced Orthopaedics at Sinai Hospital, Baltimore, Maryland

MICHAEL E. BRAGE, MD
Professor of Foot and Ankle Surgery, Department of Orthopaedic Surgery, University of Washington, Santa Monica, California

CHRISTOPHER P. CHIODO, MD
Department of Orthopedic Surgery, Brigham and Women's Hospital, Boston, Massachusetts

J. CHRIS COETZEE, MD
Twin Cities Orthopedics, Edina, Minnesota

JESSICA A. COTTRELL, PhD
Assistant Professor, Department of Biological Sciences, Seton Hall University, South Orange, New Jersey

TIMOTHY R. DANIELS, MD, FRCSC
Professor, Division of Orthopaedic Surgery, St. Michael's Hospital, University of Toronto, Toronto, Ontario, Canada

TRAVIS J. DEKKER, MD
Department of Orthopaedic Surgery, Duke University Medical Center, Durham, North Carolina

CHRISTOPHER W. DIGIOVANNI, MD
Visiting Professor and Vice Chairman (Academic Affairs); Chief, Division of Foot and Ankle Surgery, Department of Orthopaedic Surgery, Massachusetts General Hospital, Harvard Medical School, Boston, Massachusetts

ANDREW DODD, MD, FRCSC
Division of Orthopaedic Surgery, St. Michael's Hospital, University of Toronto, Toronto, Ontario, Canada

MARK GLAZEBROOK, MSc, PhD, Dip Sports Med, MD, FRCS(C)
Orthopaedic Surgeon and Researcher Subspecialty, Reconstructive Foot & Ankle Surgery & Orthopaedic Sports Medicine, Queen Elizabeth II Health Sciences Center; Associate Professor, Dalhousie University, Halifax, Nova Scotia, Canada

JOSHUA S. HARFORD, MS
Department of Orthopaedic Surgery, Duke University Medical Center, Durham, North Carolina

JEREMY HREHA, MD
Department of Orthopaedics, Rutgers New Jersey Medical School, Newark, New Jersey

JOHN G. KENNEDY, MD, MCh, MMSc, FRCS (Orth)
The Foot & Ankle Service, Hospital for Special Surgery, New York, New York

ETHAN S. KRELL, MBS
Medical Student & Research Fellow, Department of Orthopaedics, Rutgers New Jersey Medical School, Newark, New Jersey

SHELDON S. LIN, MD
Associate Professor, Department of Orthopaedics, Rutgers New Jersey Medical School, Doctor's Office Center, Newark, New Jersey

THEODORE I. MALININ, MD
Professor, Department of Orthopaedic Surgery, University of Miami Miller School of Medicine, Miami, Florida

MICHELE MARCOLONGO, PhD
Department Head and Professor, Department of Materials Science and Engineering, Materials Science and Engineering, Drexel University, Philadelphia, Pennsylvania

CHRISTOPHER P. MILLER, MD
Carl J. Shapiro Department of Orthopaedics, Beth Israel Deaconess Medical Center, Boston, Massachusetts

HARVEY E. MONTIJO, MD
Department of Orthopedics, University of British Columbia, Vancouver, British Columbia, Canada

MARK S. MYERSON, MD
Medical Director, The Foot and Ankle Association, Inc.; Institute for Foot and Ankle Recon at Mercy, Baltimore, Maryland

J. PATRICK O'CONNOR, PhD
Associate Professor, Department of Orthopaedics, Rutgers-New Jersey Medical School, Newark, New Jersey

MURRAY PENNER, MD, FRCSC
Clinical Professor, Department of Orthopedics, University of British Columbia, Vancouver, British Columbia, Canada

ANDREW W. ROSS, BA
The Foot & Ankle Service, Hospital for Special Surgery, New York, New York

LEW C. SCHON, MD
Editor, Department of Orthopaedic Surgery, MedStar Union Memorial Hospital, Baltimore, Maryland

ERIC W. TAN, MD
Department of Orthopaedic Surgery, Keck School of Medicine, University of Southern California, Los Angeles, California

H. THOMAS TEMPLE, MD
Senior Vice President for Translational Research and Economic Development; Professor, Orthopaedic Surgery, Nova Southeastern University, Fort Lauderdale, Florida

JESSICA CARDENAS TURNER, MS, PhD Candidate
Department of Biomedical Engineering, New Jersey Institute of Technology, Newark, New Jersey

PETER WHITE, MD
Department of Orthopaedic Surgery, Duke University Medical Center, Durham, North Carolina

JOAN R. WILLIAMS, MD
Associate Professor of Foot and Ankle Surgery, University of California Los Angeles Department of Orthopaedic Surgery, Santa Monica, California

YOUICHI YASUI, MD
The Foot & Ankle Service, Hospital for Special Surgery, New York, New York; Department of Orthopaedic Surgery, Teikyo University School of Medicine, Tokyo, Japan

MICHAEL G. YERANOSIAN, MD
Department of Orthopaedics, Rutgers New Jersey Medical School, Newark, New Jersey

DIANA S. YOUNG, BSc, MD, FRCS(C)
Reconstructive Foot & Ankle Surgery & Orthopaedic Sports Medicine, Queen Elizabeth II Health Sciences Center, Dalhousie University, Halifax, Nova Scotia, Canada

ALISTAIR YOUNGER, MD, FRCSC
Professor, Department of Orthopedics, University of British Columbia, Vancouver, British Columbia, Canada

Contributors

MARK S. MYERSON, MD
Medical Director, The Foot and Ankle Association, Inc., Institute for Foot and Ankle Reconstruction at Mercy, Baltimore, Maryland

J. PATRICK O'CONNOR, PhD
Associate Professor, Department of Orthopaedics, Rutgers New Jersey Medical School, Newark, New Jersey

MURRAY PENNER, MD, FRCSC
Clinical Professor, Department of Orthopaedics, University of British Columbia, Vancouver, British Columbia, Canada

LEW C. SCHON, MD
Director, Department of Orthopaedic Surgery, MedStar Union Memorial Hospital, Baltimore, Maryland

ERIC W. TAN, MD
Department of Orthopaedic Surgery, Keck School of Medicine, University of Southern California, Los Angeles, California

R. THOMAS TEMPLE, MD
Senior Vice President for Translational Research and Economic Development, Professor, Orthopaedic Surgery, Nova Southeastern University, Fort Lauderdale, Florida

JESSICA GANCORMAS TURNER, MS, PhD Candidate
Department of Biomedical Engineering, New Jersey Institute of Technology, Newark, New Jersey

PETER WHITE, MD
Department of Orthopaedic Surgery, Dalhousie University Medical Center, Halifax, Nova Scotia, Canada

NOAH R. WILLIAMS, MD
Associate Professor of Foot and Ankle Surgery, University of California, Los Angeles; Department of Orthopaedic Surgery, Santa Monica, California

YOUICHI YASUI, MD
Hospital for Special Surgery, New York, New York; Department of Orthopaedic Surgery, Teikyo University School of Medicine, Tokyo, Japan

MICHAEL G. YERANOSIAN, MD
Department of Orthopaedic Surgery, New Jersey Medical School, Newark, New Jersey

DIANA S. YOUNG, BSc, MD, FRCS(C)
Department of Foot & Ankle Surgery & Orthopaedic Surgery, Queen Elizabeth II Health Science Center, Dalhousie University, Halifax, Nova Scotia, Canada

ALISTAIR YOUNGER, MD, FRCSC
Professor, Department of Orthopaedics, University of British Columbia, Vancouver, British Columbia, Canada

Contents

Nonunion after tibial shaft fracture and hindfoot arthrodesis remains a major problem. Known risk factors include advanced age, immunosuppression, smoking, and diabetes. Several factors must be considered in the fracture healing process. This review evaluates the efficacy of orthobiologics in improving union rates after fracture or arthrodesis. Use of compounds have shown increased cellular proliferation experimentally. Percutaneous autologous bone marrow has shown increased cellular proliferation. Matrix supplementation has shown significant improvements in bone healing. Several studies have highlighted the importance of adequate graft fill over graft type. Patients at increased risk for nonunion would benefit most from these adjuvant therapies.

This review describes the normal healing process for bone, ligaments, and tendons, including primary and secondary healing as well as bone-to-bone fusion. It depicts the important mediators and cell types involved in the inflammatory, reparative, and remodeling stages of each healing process. It also describes the main challenges for clinicians when trying to repair bone, ligaments, and tendons with a specific emphasis on Charcot neuropathy, fifth metatarsal fractures, arthrodesis, and tendon sheath and adhesions. Current treatment options and research areas are also reviewed.

Nonunion remains the most impactful complication following ankle and hindfoot arthrodesis. Historically, surgeons have relied on autologous bone graft (ABG) to combat nonunion risk. Although effective, ABG remains limited in quantity, varies in quality, and can be associated with harvest site pain and morbidity. Use of alternative bone-stimulating agents, however, avoids harvesting an autograft, and provides a more predictable dose–response efficacy. This article highlights findings from basic science, animal, and human clinical research that led to the approval of Augment Bone Graft. We present an adaptation of the surgical techniques described for investigators participating in the pivotal trial.

Joint arthrodesis utilizing autogenous bone graft remains the gold standard of treatment in fusion procedures of the foot and ankle. Graft harvest, however, has been associated with increased morbidity to patients as well as increased costs. With this in mind, multiple clinical studies have evaluated the efficacy of recombinant human platelet-derived growth factor (rh-PDGF-BB) with beta-tricalcium phosphate (B-TCP) to augment in foot and ankle arthrodesis with favorable results. These factors have led to the increased use of rh-PDGF-BB with B-TCP in Vancouver with good clinical results.

Arthrodesis of the hindfoot is a common procedure for degenerative joint disease and/or severe deformity. Nonunion is a common complication from this procedure, causing an increased burden to the patient and health care system, often resulting in the need for revision surgery. Recombinant human platelet-derived growth factor (rhPDGF) has been shown to be a safe and effective tool to enhance arthrodesis rates in hindfoot surgery while avoiding the potential morbidity of bone grafting. This article provides a review of the role of rhPDGF in hindfoot fusions, and the surgical technique for performing an rhPDGF enhanced double-arthrodesis through a medial approach.

Despite advances in understanding bone healing physiology and surgical techniques, delayed union and nonunion still occur after the treatment of hindfoot arthrodesis. There is increasing appeal of bone morphogenetic proteins (BMPs) owing to the innate osteoinductive abilities of BMPs. Effective treatment with BMPs has been shown in animal studies. Human clinical studies have also shown success. The only study investigating the use of recombinant human BMP (rhBMP)-2 in hindfoot arthrodesis found a significant increase in fusion rate. Treatment is cost effective, and complications from their use remain low. rhBMP-2 is a safe and effective bone-healing adjunct in hindfoot arthrodesis surgery.

Foot and ankle fusion procedures often incorporate autogenous bone graft to help achieve bony union. Pain and morbidity associated with graft harvest have resulted in decreased autograft use as alternative bone graft substitutes have become available. Recently B2A peptide-coated ceramic granules have been developed and investigated. B2A, a bioactive synthetic multi-domain peptide acting on bone morphogenetic protein receptors of osteoblast precursor cells, amplifies the cell response to bone morphogenetic proteins. Use of B2A-granule has the additional benefit of eliminating autogenous bone graft donor site morbidity. The surgical technique of subtalar arthrodesis incorporating B2A-granule is described.

Judith F. Baumhauer and Michele Marcolongo

Various methods of repairing damaged articular cartilage surfaces have been proposed, and a variety of implant materials have been tried in an attempt to decrease pain and improve function after cartilage repair. The hydrogel made of polyvinyl alcohol and saline is a unique material used as an implant in the great toe for advanced stage arthritis.

Judith F. Baumhauer and Michele Marcolongo

One of the areas of foot and ankle surgery that has had particular attention over the last 5 years has been forefoot surgery. Common procedures include correction of the lessor metatarsophalangeal joints and hammertoe deformities, specifically metatarsal shortening osteotomies and proximal interphalangeal joint fusions. The goals of these surgeries are to improve patient function and allow patients to fit into shoes more comfortably in metatarsal shortening and hammertoe.

FOOT AND ANKLE CLINICS

THE CLINICS ARE NOW AVAILABLE ONLINE!
Access your subscription at:
www.theclinics.com

Preface

Orthobiologic in Foot Ankle

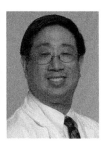

Sheldon S. Lin, MD
Editor

Significant advances continue to be made in the field of foot and ankle; especially in the treatment of arthrodesis and fracture healing, specifically addressing the complications of delayed union and nonunion. The triad concept of cellularity, critical growth factors, and matrix augmentation has ushered in a new clinical era and excitement. Despite these advances, we continue to see nonunion rates after elective arthrodesis between 7% and 10%, and of the estimated 8 million fractures in the United States, 5% to 10% continue to have issues in healing.

This Orthobiologic collection of articles is a cutting-edge preview of biological-driven concepts for the treatment of foot and ankle challenges, such as arthrodesis and their complications. Initial concepts of the topic are generally reviewed in regards to the triad of bone healing, cartilage and tendon issues, and clinical options.

The second section of this issue focuses on the new advances of critical growth factors affecting foot and ankle arthrodesis. We explore the recent FDA trial of recombinant human platelet-derived growth factor (rhPDGF), the Vancouver experience of rhPDGF, as well as the novel carrier application of PDGF. In addition, we learn of two distinct centers' experiences of rhBMP and b2A, with foot and ankle arthrodesis.

The third section of this issue focuses on the new advances of cellularity on foot and ankle abnormality, with a general review article, and the application of bone marrow. Another critical issue is to investigate the effect of the site of bone graft harvesting. This is followed by specific experiences, such as its bone marrow use in large bulk allograft and different allograft stem cells on arthrodesis. We also look at the novel application of stem cell with suture-loaded mesenchymal stem cells for its potential application in tendon healing. Finally, another article focuses on the use of platelet-rich plasma in osteochondral lesion of talus.

The final section addresses the alternative application of novel Orthobiocomposite for the treatment of hallux rigidus as well as novel plate and hammertoe design.

I have always felt that "we sit on the shoulder of giants who came before us." Clearly, this never-ending story will continue in the years to come, but I want to thank each and

Foot Ankle Clin N Am 21 (2016) xiii–xiv
http://dx.doi.org/10.1016/j.fcl.2016.09.001
1083-7515/16/© 2016 Published by Elsevier Inc.
foot.theclinics.com

every author for their effort. This compendium reflects the constant foray, diligence, and critical thinking of clinician scientists, using novel biological concepts to advance the field of foot and ankle.

Sheldon S. Lin, MD
Rutgers New Jersey Medical School
Department of Orthopaedics
Suite 7300, Doctor's Office Center
90 Bergen Street
Newark, NJ 07101-1709, USA

E-mail address:
linsheldon2@gmail.com

The Role of Orthobiologics in Fracture Healing and Arthrodesis

Sheldon S. Lin, MD[a],*, Michael G. Yeranosian, MD[b]

KEYWORDS

- Orthobiologics • Hindfoot • Fusion • Nonunion • Arthrodesis • Fracture
- Growth factors

KEY POINTS

- Use of compounds like platelet-rich plasma (PRP), mesenchymal stem cells (MSC), and recombinant human bone morphogenic protein 2 (rhBMP-2) have shown increased cellular proliferation experimentally.
- Administration of PRP has been shown to increase levels of important growth factors experimentally.
- The use of rhPDGF-BB/beta-tricalcium phosphate has shown equivalent union rates compared with autograft use after hindfoot fusions.
- Matrix supplementation with adjuvants such as MSCs and rhBMP-2 has shown significant improvements in bone healing experimentally.
- Patients at increased risk for nonunion, such as diabetics and the elderly, would likely benefit most from orthobiologic therapies.

INTRODUCTION

Nonunion after fractures and hindfoot arthrodesis remains a problem within orthopedics. After intramedullary fixation, the incidence of tibial shaft nonunion ranges from 2.4% to 2.6% for closed fractures, and up to 14.2% for open fractures.[1–5] Hindfoot fusions, meanwhile, demonstrate approximately 10% nonunion rates.[6] Improving union rates requires not only requires refinements in technique, but also an understanding and application of biological fracture healing concepts.

Fracture healing is a complex biological process involving interactions between mesenchymal stem cells (MSC), local inflammatory cytokines, and mechanical stimuli.

The authors have nothing to disclose.
[a] Department of Orthopaedics, Rutgers New Jersey Medical School, 90 Bergen Street, Room 7300, Newark, NJ 07101, USA; [b] Department of Orthopaedics, Rutgers New Jersey Medical School, 140 Bergen Street, ACC Building, Suite D-1610, Newark, NJ 07103, USA
* Corresponding author.
E-mail address: Linsheldon2@gmail.com

Initial fracture union is followed by continuous remodeling that restores the bone to its prefracture strength. The classic model of fracture healing is endochondral ossification, whereby a cartilaginous template is first formed to provide initial stability, and then replaced with bone.

Immediately after a fracture, a hematoma forms consisting of peripheral and intramedullary blood containing MSCs. The injury initiates a local inflammatory response, causing paracrine release of various cytokines. These cytokines have a wide range of effects, including chemotaxis, mitogenesis, production of vascular endothelial growth factor (VEGF), and angiogenesis. The hematoma coagulates around the fracture ends and within the medullary canal, forming a scaffold for callus formation.[7] MSCs within the hematoma, under the control of local growth factors, undergo chondrocytic differentiation, proliferation, and hypertrophy. Deposition of chondroid matrix forms a cartilaginous soft callus, provisionally stabilizing the fracture. The chondrocytes then calcify and undergo apoptosis. This initiates vascular infiltration, which facilitates osteoblast migration from the periosteum into the periphery of the soft callus. The cartilaginous template is then replaced by a hard callus composed of woven bone. Subsequent remodeling via the concerted action of osteoblasts and osteoclasts converts woven bone into mature, lamellar bone, thereby completing the healing process.

As delineated, bone healing requires an influx of progenitor cells, local growth factors to promote differentiation and proliferation, and matrix deposition to provide structural integrity and scaffolding for further bone formation. Understanding this biology has opened the door for researchers to elucidate the potential efficacy of MSCs, growth factors, and matrix substitutes—broadly termed, orthobiologics—as adjuvants to conventional treatment methods. Numerous studies have investigated the effects of these adjuvants in animal models and clinical settings. This review examines the existing data and evaluates the role of orthobiologics in achieving bony union after fracture or arthrodesis.

CELLULARITY

Cellularity at the fracture site is a sine qua non for healing, because it indicates the presence of fibroblasts, chondroblasts, and osteogenic precursors necessary for callus formation and bony union. The link between cellularity and healing has been demonstrated experimentally in a diabetic fracture model in rats. Gandhi and colleagues[8] showed that cellularity in the diabetic fracture callus was significantly less than in nondiabetic controls (34% and 42% less at days 2 and 4 after fracture, respectively). This reduction in cellularity was associated with decreased torsional rigidity ($\leq75\%$), torque to failure, and maximum shear strength in the diabetic group. In a concurrent study, Beam and colleagues[9] showed that, compared with nondiabetic controls, diabetic rats exhibited 50% and 40% decreased cell proliferation at days 2 and 4 after fracture, respectively, and a 70% reduction in torque to failure at 6 weeks. These findings suggest that systemic diseases associated with decreased cellular proliferation can impair healing after fracture.

Therapeutic use of orthobiologics to promote increased cellularity has been described in the literature. Examples of such adjuncts include platelet-rich plasma (PRP), platelet-derived growth factor (PDGF), low-dose insulin, MSCs, and recombinant human bone morphogenic protein 2 (rhBMP-2). Although randomized controlled trials have not been performed, numerous level II studies in animals have shown promise.

Gandhi and colleagues[8] demonstrated that percutaneous delivery of PRP into the fracture site of diabetic rats increased cell proliferation by 36% and torsional rigidity by 56% 2 days after fracture compared with noninjected controls. This finding may be attributed to impaired levels of expression of PDGF in the setting of diabetes. Another study in diabetic rats showed that low-dose insulin therapy increased cell proliferation by 43% and torque to failure by 61% 2 days after fracture.[9] Breitbart and colleagues[10] investigated the use of MSCs in BB Wistar rats and found significant increases in mature bone on histology at 4 and 8 weeks. In addition, they showed significantly greater endosteal bone formation, defect-filling bone formation, and total bone formation at 4 weeks compared with nontreated controls.

The usefulness of increasing fracture site cellularity with the use of orthobiologics has also been borne out clinically. Hernigou and colleagues[11] investigated the use of percutaneous autologous bone marrow grafting for aseptic, atrophic nonunions of the tibial diaphysis. Concentrated bone marrow containing progenitor cells was injected into the fracture site in 60 patients, with the assumption that injected cells would remain in situ and increase local cellularity. Fifty-three (88%) went on to union. In the 7 refractory nonunions (12%), it was found that the concentration and the total number of injected cells were significantly lower than in the group that eventually healed. This suggests a possible dose–response relationship, lending further credence to the association between cellularity and healing potential.

LOCAL GROWTH FACTORS AND CYTOKINES

Growth factors and cytokines have chemotactic and mitogenic properties, directing the migration, differentiation, and proliferation of MSCs. Many of these factors are stored in circulating platelets, which degranulate after becoming entrapped in a fibrin clot at the fracture site. Examples include PDGF-AB, transforming growth factor (TGF)-β1, insulinlike growth factor-1 (IGF-1), and VEGF.

In a level II study, Gandhi and colleagues[8] revealed the relative paucity of these growth factors at fracture sites in the previously described diabetic rat model of impaired fracture healing. At day 4 after fracture, PDGF-AB levels were reduced by 56%, TGF-β1 by 53%, IGF-1 by 61%, and VEGF by 20% compared with nondiabetic rats. At day 7, PDGF-AB levels were reduced by 45%, TGF-β1 by 50%, IGF-1 by 52%, and VEGF 54% compared with nondiabetics.

Clinical data also suggest a correlation between growth factor levels and bone healing capacity. A level III prospective comparison study by Street and colleagues[12] found decreased PDGF levels in the fracture hematoma of patients older than 75 years (5066 ± 678 pg/mL) compared with patients younger than 40 (7098 ± 650 pg/mL; $P<.01$). In another level III study, Verma and colleagues[13] demonstrated 70% decreased PDGF levels and 44% decreased VEGF levels in diabetic patients who went on to nonunion after hindfoot fusion (n = 3) compared with those that successfully fused (n = 7).

PDGF seems to be of particular importance. It functions in an autocrine feedback loop, stimulating production and release of other growth factors and cytokines. In addition to increasing cell migration and proliferation, PDGF facilitates cellular interactions with VEGF, thereby promoting neovascularization at the fracture site. A level II study by Tyndall and colleagues[14] correlated decreased PDGF levels to decreased cell proliferation. At 4 days after fracture, diabetic rats expressed 75% less PDGF microRNA compared with nondiabetic controls, with a concomitant decrease in fracture site cellularity. The association between decreased cellularity and impaired fracture healing may, therefore, be rooted in diminished expression of PDGF.

Numerous studies have investigated the effect of orthobiologics on local growth factor concentrations. Gandhi and colleagues[8] injected PRP at fracture sites in diabetic rats to and found a 4-fold increase in PDGF, a 3-fold increase in TGF-β1, a 3-fold increase in VEGF, and a 1.5-fold increase in IGF-I expression. In a concurrent level II study in diabetic rats, Al-Zube and associates[15] demonstrated that low doses of recombinant human PDGF-BB (rhPDGF-BB) increased the release of local growth factors at fracture sites compared with controls. They demonstrated increased early cellularity and improved callus biomechanical properties, including maximum torque to failure ($P = .028$) and maximum torsional rigidity ($P = .08$). Additionally, rhPDGF-BB promoted new blood vessel formation through the up-regulation of VEGF and the stabilization of new capillaries by mural cells.

Clinical studies have shown similar results. In a level I study, DiGiovanni and co-workers[16] compared rhPDGF-BB homodimer combined with an osteoconductive matrix (beta-tricalcium phosphate [β-TCP]) to autograft in patients requiring ankle or hindfoot arthrodesis. Successful union, defined as greater than 50% bone bridging on computed tomography (CT) scan, occurred in 36.9% of patients in the rhPDGF-BB/β-TCP group and 36.5% of those in the autograft group with use of the full-complement analysis ($P = .020$); and 48.5% of the rhPDGF-BB/β-TCP group and 44.3% of the autograft group with use of the all-joints analysis ($P<.001$).[16] In a parallel experiment, DiGiovanni and colleagues[17] also showed that the rate of therapeutic failures (delayed union or nonunion requiring surgery or further therapeutic intervention) was 7.3% for rhPDGF–BB/β-TCP patients and 8% for autograft patients. The authors concluded that rhPDGF-BB/β-TCP was a safe and effective alternative to autograft, without the associated donor site morbidity.

BMPs comprise a subclass of the TGF-β superfamily. Their osteoinductive properties have spurred interest in their use as adjuvants to bone healing. Azad and colleagues[18] investigated the use of recombinant human BMP-2 (rhBMP-2) in a diabetic rat segmental defect model. They found significant increases in bone formation on histology at the 3-week and 6-week time points, and increased radiographic healing at 6 weeks in the experimental group compared with the control group. Furthermore, PECAM-1 staining revealed significant increases in mean number of vessels in rhBMP-2–treated rats. Mechanical testing of the specimens at the 9-week mark demonstrated significantly greater torque to failure and torsional rigidity values in the experimental group as well.

BMP is approved currently only for use in lumbar fusions and tibial nonunions, although off-label use for ankle and hindfoot fusions has also been described. Bibbo and colleagues[19] reported the results of 112 fusions supplemented with rhBMP-2 in high-risk patients, including smokers, diabetics, and patients with a history of high-energy trauma or talar avascular necrosis. A 96% overall union rate was achieved at a mean of 11 weeks with a low rate of complications. The authors concluded rhBMP-2 was effective adjunct for bone healing in populations at high risk for nonunion.

The implications of these data are that local growth factor deficiency may contribute to nonunion after fracture or arthrodesis in certain high-risk populations. Elderly and diabetic patients may perhaps benefit most from growth factor augmentation. More level I studies are clearly warranted to shed further light on this important question.

MATRIX DEFICIENCY

The extracellular matrix of bone consists largely of hydroxyapatite and collagen, which provide structural integrity as well as a scaffold for the adherence and migration of osteogenic precursors. This scaffolding, or osteoconductive property of bone matrix, becomes especially important when larger gaps exist between healing bone ends.

Critically sized bone defects may become atrophic and scarred rather than regenerate, leading to nonunion.[20] Matrix also provides the medium through which embedded osteocytes, via branching canaliculi, communicate mechanosensory stimuli and control bone remodeling.[21–24] Disruption of matrix therefore also interrupts the intercellular signaling necessary for normal healing to occur.[25] The use of supplementary matrix—including autograft, allograft, and synthetic matrix substitutes—to bridge critical defects and improve union rates has been investigated both experimentally and clinically.

Matrix deficiency is recreated experimentally by producing critical defects, typically greater than 1.5 times the cross-sectional diameter in a region of bone.[26,27] This model has been used in numerous studies in rats, which show significant nonunion rates after creation of such defects.[18,26,28–30] Additionally, multiple studies investigating the use of supplementary matrix with adjuvants such as MSCs and rhBMP-2 in diabetic rats have shown significant improvements in bone healing.[10,18]

Nonunion rates of about 10% continue to be reported after ankle and hindfoot arthrodesis.[6] Several clinical studies have investigated the effects of bone graft and matrix substitutes on fusion rates after these procedures.[6,16,31] A level III study by McGarvey and Braly[31] compared the use of allograft versus autograft in 41 hindfoot arthrodeses, and found union rates of 87.5% and 94.2% with allograft and autograft, respectively. DiGiovanni and associates[16] investigated the use of rhPDGF–BB/β-TCP, showing comparable healing at 52 weeks between the rhPDGF-BB/β-TCP group (88.3%) and autograft group (87.2%, level II). Thordarson and Kuehn[6] compared the use of 2 different demineralized bone graft products and showed no difference in efficacy between the 2 grafts, and no improvement in union rates compared with historical controls (level III). A recent logistic regression analysis of 159 studies providing data from foot and ankle arthrodesis surgery found a trend toward higher union rates with autograft compared with no graft.[32]

In addition to graft type, a variable to consider is the completeness of defect bridging with graft material. Digiovanni and coworkers[33] investigated the effect of adequate versus inadequate bone graft fill and autograft versus rhPDGF-BB/β-TCP on fusion rates after ankle/hindfoot arthrodesis in 411 patients across 37 institutions. Adequate graft fill was defined as graft occupying greater than 50% of the cross-sectional area of the fusion space on the 9-week CT scan, and fusion was defined as greater than 50% osseous bridging on the 24-week CT scan. With both autograft and rhPDGF-BB/β-TCP, fusion rates were significantly higher in joints with adequate fill (82% vs 21%; $P<.0001$; level II). Furthermore, Glazebrook and colleagues[34] demonstrated that greater than 25% to 49% of trabecular bridging on CT scans resulted in a clinically successful fusion (level IV).

The importance of sufficient matrix is highlighted by the difficulty to heal critical defects without matrix supplementation. Data in the current literature emphasize the importance of sufficient graft fill rather than the superiority of 1 graft type over another. There is a lack of high-quality, randomized controlled trials investigating this topic, however, because most data come from level II, III, or IV studies. Furthermore, a relatively unaddressed topic is the role of allogeneic grafts.

Case #1
___

A 67-year-old man has severe ankle arthritis. Standing ankle radiographs demonstrated joint space narrowing, malalignment, and osteophyte formation (**Fig. 1**). He underwent tibiotalar fusion augmented with rhPDGF–BB/β-TCP bone graft substitute. Postoperative radiographs and a sagittal CT image at 24 weeks are shown in **Figs. 2** and **3**, respectively, demonstrating extensive bony bridging. Radiographs at

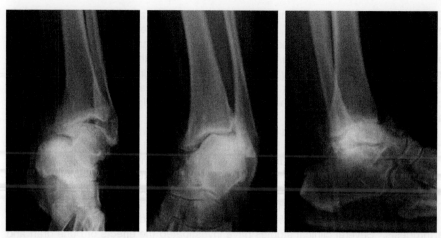

Fig. 1. Anteroposterior, Mortise, and lateral views demonstrate severe tibiotalar joint asymmetry with severe arthritis.

52 weeks demonstrate complete fusion (**Fig. 4**). Clinically, the patient was doing very well, with markedly decreased pain with ambulation.

Case #2

A 30-year-old man underwent a triple arthrodesis procedure with no evidence of union 1 year postoperatively. Radiographs are shown in **Fig. 5**. The patient then underwent revision triple arthrodesis supplemented with a commercial PRP product. Successful union was achieved by the 6-week mark (**Fig. 6**). Pain improved significantly, and the patient was satisfied with the outcome.

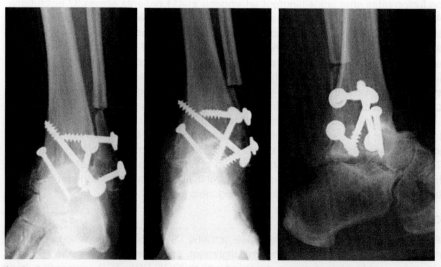

Fig. 2. Anteroposterior, Mortise, and lateral views demonstrate successful ankle arthrodesis with fibula onlay technique, with screw fixation and recombinant human platelet-derived growth factor-BB– beta-tricalcium phosphate at 6 months after surgery.

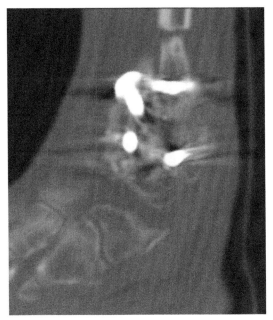

Fig. 3. Sagittal section computed tomography scan shows bone bridging of ankle fusion site at 6 months after surgery.

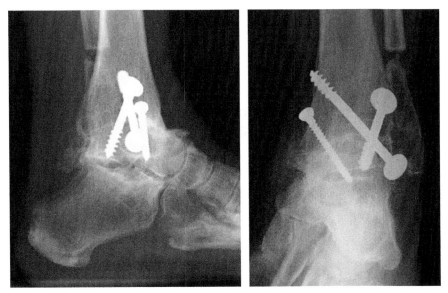

Fig. 4. Anteroposterior and lateral views of the left ankle shows successful ankle arthrodesis at 1 year after surgery.

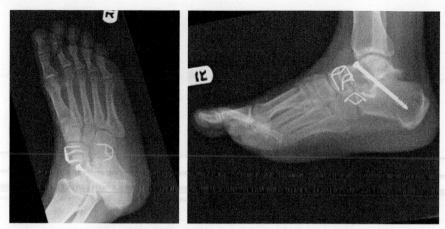

Fig. 5. Anteroposterior and lateral views of the right foot reveals nonunion after an attempted triple arthrodesis of right foot.

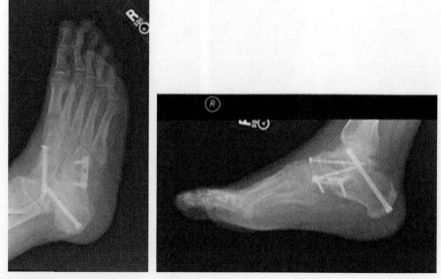

Fig. 6. Anteroposterior and lateral views of the right foot demonstrated successful revision of triple with new hardware and platelet-rich plasma.

SUMMARY

Understanding of the role of cellularity, growth factors, and matrix deficiency in bone healing is critical to the application of various adjuvant therapies to decrease nonunion rates. Bone marrow grafting has been shown to improve tibial nonunion rates clinically. Because both diabetic and elderly patients have been shown to have deficient levels of PDGF and VEGF, use of rhPDGF-BB may be particularly useful in these high-risk populations. Administration of PRP has been shown to increase levels of important growth factors PDGF-AB, TGF-B, IGF-I, and VEGF experimentally, whereas rhPDGF-BB/ß-TCP has shown similar benefits both experimentally and clinically in hindfoot fusions. With regard to matrix deficiency, the importance of adequate graft fill seems to be more important than the graft type used in achieving union.

ACKNOWLEDGMENTS

The authors acknowledge that considerable work was done on this article by the following individuals: Augustine Tawadros, BA, Department of Orthopedics, Rutgers New Jersey Medical School, Newark, New Jersey and Joseph A. Ippolito, BA, Department of Orthopedics Rutgers New Jersey Medical School, Newark, New Jersey.

REFERENCES

1. Antonova E, Le TK, Burge R, et al. Tibia shaft fractures: costly burden of nonunions. BMC Musculoskelet Disord 2013;14:42.
2. Drosos GI, Bishay M, Karnezis IA, et al. Factors affecting fracture healing after intramedullary nailing of the tibial diaphysis for closed and grade I open fractures. J Bone Joint Surg Br 2006;88(2):227–31.
3. Gaebler C, Berger U, Schandelmaier P, et al. Rates and odds ratios for complications in closed and open tibial fractures treated with unreamed, small diameter tibial nails: a multicenter analysis of 467 cases. J Orthop Trauma 2001;15(6):415–23.
4. Malik MH, Harwood P, Diggle P, et al. Factors affecting rates of infection and nonunion in intramedullary nailing. J Bone Joint Surg Br 2004;86(4):556–60.
5. Sledge SL, Johnson KD, Henley MB, et al. Intramedullary nailing with reaming to treat non-union of the tibia. J Bone Joint Surg Am 1989;71(7):1004–19.
6. Thordarson DB, Kuehn S. Use of demineralized bone matrix in ankle/hindfoot fusion. Foot Ankle Int 2003;24(7):557–60.
7. Marsell R, Einhorn TA. The biology of fracture healing. Injury 2011;42(6):551–5.
8. Gandhi A, Doumas C, Dumas C, et al. The effects of local platelet rich plasma delivery on diabetic fracture healing. Bone 2006;38(4):540–6.
9. Beam HA, Parsons JR, Lin SS. The effects of blood glucose control upon fracture healing in the BB Wistar rat with diabetes mellitus. J Orthop Res 2002;20(6):1210–6.
10. Breitbart EA, Meade S, Azad V, et al. Mesenchymal stem cells accelerate bone allograft incorporation in the presence of diabetes mellitus. J Orthop Res 2010;28(7):942–9.
11. Hernigou P, Poignard A, Beaujean F, et al. Percutaneous autologous bone-marrow grafting for nonunions. Influence of the number and concentration of progenitor cells. J Bone Joint Surg Am 2005;87(7):1430–7.
12. Street JT, Wang JH, Wu QD, et al. The angiogenic response to skeletal injury is preserved in the elderly. J Orthop Res 2001;19(6):1057–66.

13. Verma RA, Koerner JA, Breitbart EA, et al. Correlation of growth factor levels at the fusion site of diabetic patients undergoing hindfoot arthrodesis and clinical outcome. Curr Orthop Pract 2011;22(3):251–6.

14. Tyndall WA, Beam HA, Zarro C, et al. Decreased platelet derived growth factor expression during fracture healing in diabetic animals. Clin Orthop Relat Res 2003;(408):319–30.

15. Al-Zube L, Breitbart EA, O'Connor JP, et al. Recombinant human platelet-derived growth factor BB (rhPDGF-BB) and beta-tricalcium phosphate/collagen matrix enhance fracture healing in a diabetic rat model. J Orthop Res 2009;27(8):1074–81.

16. DiGiovanni CW, Lin SS, Baumhauer JF, et al. Recombinant human platelet-derived growth factor-BB and beta-tricalcium phosphate (rhPDGF-BB/β-TCP): an alternative to autogenous bone graft. J Bone Joint Surg Am 2013;95(13):1184–92.

17. DiGiovanni CW, Lin S, Pinzur M. Recombinant human PDGF-BB in foot and ankle fusion. Expert Rev Med Devices 2012;9(2):111–22.

18. Azad V, Breitbart E, Al-Zube L, et al. rhBMP-2 enhances the bone healing response in a diabetic rat segmental defect model. J Orthop Trauma 2009;23(4):267–76.

19. Bibbo C, Patel DV, Haskell MD. Recombinant bone morphogenetic protein-2 (rhBMP-2) in high-risk ankle and hindfoot fusions. Foot Ankle Int 2009;30(7):597–603.

20. Langer R, Vacanti JP. Tissue engineering. Science 1993;260(5110):920–6.

21. Beaupré GS, Orr TE, Carter DR. An approach for time-dependent bone modeling and remodeling–theoretical development. J Orthop Res 1990;8(5):651–61.

22. Cowin SC, Hegedus DH. Bone remodeling I: theory of adaptive elasticity. J Elasticity 1976;6(3):313–26.

23. Hart RT, Davy DT, Heiple KG. A computational method for stress analysis of adaptive elastic materials with a view toward applications in strain-induced bone remodeling. J Biomech Eng 1984;106(4):342–50.

24. Weinans H, Huiskes R, Grootenboer HJ. The behavior of adaptive bone-remodeling simulation models. J Biomech 1992;25(12):1425–41.

25. Doblaré M, García JM, Gómez MJ. Modelling bone tissue fracture and healing: a review. Eng Fract Mech 2004;71(13–14):1809–40.

26. Einhorn TA, Lane JM, Burstein AH, et al. The healing of segmental bone defects induced by demineralized bone matrix. A radiographic and biomechanical study. J Bone Joint Surg Am 1984;66(2):274–9.

27. Key JA. The effect of a local calcium depot on osteogenesis and healing of fractures. J Bone Joint Surg 1934;16(1):176–84.

28. Feighan JE, Davy D, Prewett AB, et al. Induction of bone by a demineralized bone matrix gel: a study in a rat femoral defect model. J Orthop Res 1995;13(6):881–91.

29. Hunt TR, Schwappach JR, Anderson HC. Healing of a segmental defect in the rat femur with use of an extract from a cultured human osteosarcoma cell-line (Saos-2). A preliminary report. J Bone Joint Surg Am 1996;78(1):41–8.

30. Nottebaert M, Lane JM, Juhn A, et al. Omental angiogenic lipid fraction and bone repair. An experimental study in the rat. J Orthop Res 1989;7(2):157–69.

31. McGarvey WC, Braly WG. Bone graft in hindfoot arthrodesis: allograft vs autograft. Orthopedics 1996;19(5):389–94.

32. Lareau CR, Deren ME, Fantry A, et al. Does autogenous bone graft work? A logistic regression analysis of data from 159 papers in the foot and ankle literature. Foot Ankle Surg 2015;21(3):150–9.

33. DiGiovanni CW, Lin S, Daniels T, et al. The importance of sufficient graft material in achieving a critical foot or ankle fusion Mass. J Bone Joint Surg Am 2016; 98(15):1260–7.
34. Glazebrook M, Beasley W, Daniels T, et al. Establishing the relationship between clinical outcome and extent of osseous bridging between computed tomography assessment in isolated hindfoot and ankle fusions. Foot Ankle Int 2013;34(12): 1612–8.

The Biology of Bone and Ligament Healing

Jessica A. Cottrell, PhD[a],*, Jessica Cardenas Turner, MS, PhD[b],
Treena Livingston Arinzeh, PhD[b], J. Patrick O'Connor, PhD[c]

KEYWORDS

- Bone fracture healing • Tendon and ligament healing • Arthrodesis
- Tissue regeneration • Wound healing • Charcot neuropathy
- Fifth metatarsal fractures

KEY POINTS

- Bone healing occurs through primary or secondary ossification to restore the functional integrity of the affected bone.
- Charcot neuropathy and certain fifth metatarsal fractures have poor healing success rates that are exacerbated by specific risk factors and comorbidities.
- Ligament and tendon healing is not a regenerative process but occurs through a distinct wound healing process that requires short-term fibrocartilage formation and long-term tissue remodeling to restore function.

INTRODUCTION

Foot and ankle function relies on bones, ligaments, and tendons (BLT) for strength, support, and movement. Injuries to these lower extremities occur frequently at work or during sport-related activities and still account for more than 20% of all emergency department visits annually.[1] Foot and ankle injuries are common in patients between 20 and 60 years old and frequently include ligament and bone. Trauma care has made

Disclosure Statement: Dr T.L. Arinzeh receives research funding from the Department of Defense (W81XWH-14-1-0482), National Science Foundation, Musculoskeletal Transplant Foundation (Treena Arinzeh's grant), New Jersey Commission on Spinal Cord Research(CSCR16ERG014), Christopher L. Moseley Foundation, and Integra LifeSciences, Inc. Dr J.P. O'Connor is an owner of Accelalox Inc, which is developing novel therapies to promote bone regeneration, and receives research funding from the Musculoskeletal Transplant Foundation and the National Institutes of Health. Dr J.A. Cottrell have nothing to disclose. Dr J.C. Turner receives research funding from National Aeronautics and Space Administration Fellowship (NNX13AL56H).
 a Department of Biological Sciences, Seton Hall University, 400 South Orange Avenue, South Orange, NJ 07101, USA; b Department of Biomedical Engineering, New Jersey Institute of Technology, 323 Martin Luther King Boulevard, Newark, NJ 07102, USA; c Department of Orthopaedics, Rutgers-New Jersey Medical School, Medical Sciences Building, Room E-659, 185 South Orange Avenue, Newark, NJ 07103, USA
* Corresponding author.
E-mail address: cottreje@shu.edu

advances over the past 3 decades, which has contributed to a steady decline in the rate of ligament injury. Despite these improvements, the rate of serious bone injury has continued to grow over this same time.[1] BLT tissue injuries trigger an inflammatory response, which stimulates synthesis of cytokines, growth factors, and other mediators to coordinate the normal tissue healing response. When BLT injuries are complex or associated with other comorbidities and risk factors, mechanical or biochemical intervention is required to help return the injured tissue back to its original strength and function. The normal mechanisms that guide BLT healing as well as current treatment challenges for these injuries are the focus of this article.

THE BIOLOGY OF BONE HEALING

Fractured bone is capable of undergoing repair and regeneration. Approximately 10% of fractures, however, result in delayed fracture healing (delayed union), malunion, or nonunion.[2] In these cases, the patients experience persistent pain and ultimately require medical intervention to promote healing of the fracture.[3,4] Fracture healing can be classified into primary and secondary healing. Primary healing requires rigid fixation because it can only occur in the complete absence of motion at the fracture site whereas secondary healing requires minimization of motion (eg, cast or splint) at the fracture site. Secondary healing benefits from limited motion at the fracture site to promote callus formation that ultimately leads to internal immobilization of the fracture. The sequence of events that takes place during fracture healing and bone development has been extensively studied at the cellular and molecular levels.[5–9] These findings have increased the level of understanding of bone healing and may further advance surgical and therapeutic strategies for promoting the repair of damaged bone. This section discusses the biology of different forms of fracture healing, with secondary healing discussed first because it is the most common form of healing, followed by an overview of bone-to-bone fusions.

Secondary Healing

Secondary healing involves endochondral (EC) ossification, which mediates the stabilization of the injury and restoration of damaged vasculature prior to regeneration of the tissue during the fracture healing process. This fracture healing process can be divided into 3 overlapping phases: (1) inflammatory, (2) reparative, and (3) remodeling, where intramembranous (IM) and EC ossification occur during the reparative phase (**Fig. 1**).[10] Various cellular components are recruited at different stages in response to growth factors and cytokines. The inflammatory phase occurs immediately after injury. In humans, the inflammatory phase lasts approximately 1 week whereas in mice, the inflammatory phase lasts less than 4 days.[11] The damaged vasculature and bone marrow facilitate the influx of primitive mesenchymal stem cells (MSCs) into the fracture site.[10] During hemostasis, platelets release transforming growth factor β (TGF-β) and platelet-derived growth factor (PDGF) for the stimulation and chemotaxis of undifferentiated MSCs and macrophages. Macrophages are initially recruited to remove debris, necrotic tissue, and pathogens at the site of injury. A recent study demonstrated that fracture healing is impaired in macrophage-depleted mice wherein EC ossification is altered.[12] Macrophages express fibroblast growth factor 1 (FGF-1) and fibroblast growth factor 2 (FGF-2), interleukin-1 (IL-1), and TGF-β during the inflammatory phase which may help promote angiogenesis within the fracture.[12] MSCs recruited from the exposed bone marrow, periosteum (outer lining), or endosteum (inner lining) differentiate into fibroblasts, chondrocytes, and osteoblasts during the reparative phase.[13]

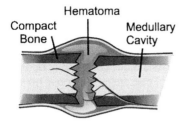

Compact Bone, Hematoma, Medullary Cavity

Inflammatory Phase—Vascular endothelial damage results in hematoma formation, complement cascade, and clotting cascade leading to the accumulation of PMNs, lymphocytes, platelets, blood monocytes, macrophages, neutrophils, osteoclasts, and undifferentiated cells. The cells express various genes including TGF-β, FGF-I, FGF-II, PDGF, IGF-I, IGF-II, BMP-2,-4,-7, osteonectin, BMPR I/II, IL-1, IL-6, and GMCSF.

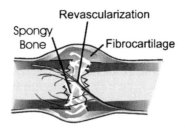

Spongy Bone, Revascularization, Fibrocartilage

Reparative Phase—(Fibrocartilage Callus Formation)- Fibrous tissue and new cartilage are beginning to form and revascularization is taking place. The appearance of macrophages, chondroblasts, chondrocytes, osteoclasts, fibroblasts, and endothelial cells is seen along with the expression of TGF-β, FGF-1, FGF-2, PDGF, IGF-I, IGF-II, BMP-2,-4,-7, osteonectin, fibronectin, BMPR I/II, smads 2,3,4, IL-1, IL-6, and collagens (II,III,IV,V,VI,IX,X).

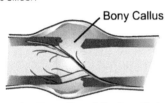

Bony Callus

Reparative Phase—(Bony Callus Formation)- Intramembranous and endochondral ossification is taking place to lay down new woven bone. The appearance of macrophages, chondroblasts, chondrocytes, osteoblasts, osteoclasts, and endothelial cells is seen along with the express ion of TGF-β, FGF-1, FGF-2, PDGF, IGF-I, IGF-II, BMP-2,-4,-7, osteonectin, osteopontin, osteocalcin, BMPR I/II, smads 2,3,4, IL-1, IL-6, and collagens (I, II, III, IV, V, VI, IX, X).

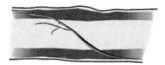

Remodeling Phase—Replacement of woven bone by lamellar bone and the resorption of excess callus. Gradual modification of the fracture region leads to restoration of normal bone architecture.

Fig. 1. Representation of fracture repair, including growth factors and cytokines at each stage. BMPR, bone morphogenetic protein receptor; GMCSF, granulocyte macrophage colony stimulating factor; MAD, mothers against decapentaplegic; PMN, polymorphonuclear leukocyte; SMA SMAD, caenorhabditis elegans protein. (*From* Sfeir C, Ho L, Doll BA, et al. Fracture repair. In: Lieberman JR, Friedlaender GE, editors. Bone regeneration and repair. Totowa (NJ): Humana Press Inc; 2005. p. 22; with permission.)

Both IM and EC ossification occur simultaneously during the reparative phase. IM ossification primarily occurs at the peripheral ends of the presumptive callus as precursor cells differentiate into osteoblasts that lay down woven bone (hard callus). These osteoblasts express TGF-β, FGF-1, and FGF-2, insulin-like growth factor I (IGF-I), and bone morphogenetic proteins (BMPs). In contrast, EC ossification requires the formation of cartilaginous intermediate tissue (soft callus) prior to ossification. Thus, EC occurs within the bulk of the fracture space where vasculature is initially limited. Within the soft callus, proliferating chondrocytes express TGF-β, IGF-I, IGF-II, BMP-2, BMP-4, and BMP-7 in association with increased collagen and cartilage matrix synthesis.[14] Chondrocytes at the IM/EC interface (chondro-osseous junction) transition into hypertrophy while increasing their cell volume as they continue to secrete cartilaginous extracellular matrix. Hypertrophy is initiated and regulated by expression of various transcription factors, primarily, *Runx2* and *Runx3*. As chondrocytes reach hypertrophy and begin to undergo nonapoptotic cell death, matrix metalloproteinases 13 and 9 are released to degrade collagen type II and aggrecan (cartilage matrix components) whereas the hypertrophic chondrocytes express IGF-II and synthesize collagen X.[14] Additionally, hypertrophy up-regulates the expression of vascular endothelial growth factor. Cartilage is highly avascular; thus, the vascular endothelial growth factor expression is crucial for vascular invasion necessary for ossification of the cartilage tissue. Along with new blood vessels, osteoclasts, osteoblasts, and bone marrow cells also invade the hypertrophic cartilage tissue from the IM/EC ossification interface. Osteoclasts partially resorb the cartilaginous matrix, whereas osteoblasts use any remaining matrix as a scaffold to deposit bone matrix. Eventually the matrix becomes mineralized as bone cells begin to deposit hydroxyapatite (inorganic mineral present in bone).[10,15] Mineralization is highly regulated by the expression of alkaline phosphatase, osteonectin (binds calcium), osteocalcin (hydroxyapatite regulator), TGF-β (increases alkaline phosphatase and osteonectin expression), and BMPs 2, 4, 7, and 9 (increase alkaline phosphatase and osteocalcin expression).[8] IL-6 is produced by osteoblasts to stimulate bone resorption, whereas IGF-II modulates resorption by osteoclasts. Eventually woven bone replaces the mineralized callus, and the remodeling phase begins.[2,10,15–17] Remodeling after fracture repair entails the replacement of woven bone with lamellar bone orchestrated by osteoprogenitor stem cells that differentiate into osteoblasts (bone forming) and osteoclasts (bone resorption). Osteopontin mediates anchoring of osteoclasts to bone matrix for resorption during remodeling.[18] Overall, the remodeling phase occurs gradually in response to mechanical loading, and can last up to several years.

Primary Healing

Primary bone healing requires rigid fixation at both ends of the fracture to ensure that the fracture site is completely immobilized, which suppresses callus formation. In primary bone healing, cells do not form fibrous or cartilaginous tissue within the fracture gap. Instead, the fracture is repaired from woven bone laid down through IM ossification. Two different types of primary bone healing exist, (1) gap healing and (2) contact healing.[16,17] In gap healing, small fracture gaps are filled with woven bone, which is then remodeled to complete healing. During remodeling, osteoclasts create cutting cones, tunnel-like cavities through the bone, and are trailed by osteoblasts that form new lamellar bone while reconstructing haversian canals and osteons.[19,20] Different from gap healing, contact healing requires the fracture fragments to be rigidly fixed in contact with each other (eg, bone fusions). Because fracture gaps are absent, osteoclasts initiate the formation of cutting cones and the reconstructions of the haversian canals and osteons immediately, without the need for woven bone deposition. Primary healing requires rigid fixation whereas secondary healing benefits from some motion within the microenvironment of the fracture site.[16,17,21]

Bone-to-Bone Fusions

Bone or joint fusions (arthrodesis) are performed surgically to relieve severe pain and restore stability at the joint (**Fig. 2**).[22,23] In bone-to-bone fusions, the surgeon completely removes the articular cartilage or fibrous tissue covering the end of the bones at the joint to fully expose the underlying bone tissue. These exposed surfaces are then compressed and held together by fixation with pins, screws, plates, or rods at an optimal position to create the fusion, which permanently limits the mobility at the joint.[24] Primary bone healing occurs where the bone surfaces are pressed into contact and held by rigid fixation. Osteoclasts and osteoblasts then begin a primary healing response, as discussed previously.[19,20] For example, the ankle is a complex hinged synovial joint consisting of portions of these 3 bones: talus, tibia, and fibula; its anatomy allows for a wide range of motion (dorsiflexion and plantar flexion, eversion, and inversion). In ankle arthrodesis, the distal tibia is typically fused to the talus, and in some cases, the fibula is included in the fusion.[23] Viable candidates for arthrodesis include patients who suffer from developmental defects, posttraumatic osteoarthritis,

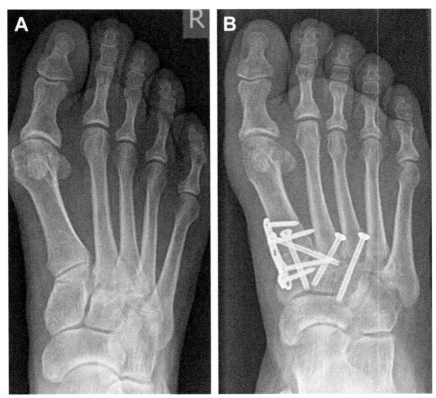

Fig. 2. (*A*) Hallux valgus deformity corrected with (*B*) arthrodesis of tarsometatarsal joints (Lapidus procedure). (*From* Gougoulias N, Lampridis V. Midfoot arthrodesis. Foot Ankle Surg 2016;22(1):23; with permission.)

rheumatoid arthritis, nonunion or poorly healed fractures, necrosis, implant/graft failure, or neuromuscular disorders, such as post poliomyelitis. Commonly reported sites for arthrodesis procedures include the ankle,[23,25–27] wrist,[28] foot,[22,29,30] sacroiliac (rarely postpartum),[31] and spine.[32–34]

Autogenous bone grafts are often used in arthrodesis, including ankle arthrodesis. Patients can benefit from osteoprogenitor cells within autogenous bone graft to augment the rate of bone fusion and reduce the risk of nonunion.[21] Different from contact healing, the process of bone graft incorporation in arthrodesis models is similar to secondary fracture healing process where inflammatory, reparative, and remodeling phases are seen.[21] Spinal arthrodesis with autogenous iliac crest bone graft remains the gold standard to relieve back pain associated with instability of the spine. Approximately 500,000 spinal arthrodesis surgeries occur per year in the United States.[33] In those joints in which immobility causes severe disability, such as the hip, cubitus (elbow), and knee joints, arthrodesis is considered only in selected patients who are not suitable candidates for preferred operative treatments (eg, total joint replacement) or after nonoperative and preferred operative treatments have failed.[35,36] In the latter, arthrodesis is generally a salvage procedure.

Complications associated with arthrodesis procedures have been reported and include a 10% to 60% rate of adjacent joint deterioration in the long term, 10% to 20% rate of nonunion, and 3% to 25% rate of postoperative infection.[25] Joint replacement (arthroplasty) has become increasingly popular over arthrodesis because it preserves mobility of the joint, diminishes pain significantly, and may decrease the risk of arthritis on the neighboring joints from elevated stress. Increased stress in neighboring joints is a drawback of arthrodesis.[26,37] Evidence shows that in 2004, ankle arthrodesis was performed 9.8 more times than total ankle arthroplasty (TAA) and by 2009 ankle arthrodesis was performed 2.3 times more than TAA.[26] A 4-year follow-up study comparing ankle arthrodesis to TAA found that patients who underwent ankle arthrodesis reported ankle osteoarthritis scores (AOS) for pain as 51.2 and for disability as 44.5, whereas patients post-TAA reported AOS for pain as 26.0 and for disability as 33.2. An AOS score of 0.0 indicates no pain or disability. Although TAA surgery resulted in significant pain relief, 40.5% of the patients within the TAA group required postoperative surgical intervention during the follow-up period compared with 21.7% in the arthrodesis group of patients.[26] Another report found that adjacent joints become arthritic after arthroplasty more than after arthrodesis during a 5-year follow-up.[27] In 2014, however, the American Orthopaedic Foot and Ankle Society endorsed TAA surgery as an established operative treatment option for patients with arthritic conditions affecting the ankle joint.[38] Total joint replacement is not an option for everyone; certain criteria, such as young age, high activity, obesity, misalignment, and history of alcohol and drug consumption, are considered risk factors for joint replacement surgery because they may lead to premature wear of implants and require several revision surgeries.[25,27] Overall, both arthrodesis and arthroplasty are widely used today to treat end-stage arthritic joints, and the selected route of operative treatment is specific to the patient depending on health risk factors, clinical history of the patient, the degree of damage, and the specific joint in need of repair.

CLINICAL CHALLENGES IN BONE HEALING

BLT provide important functions to the foot and ankle. When these tissues are injured, inflammation occurs followed by a highly ordered and complex process that promotes healing. Many BLT injuries, such as ankle sprains and osteochondral lesions, can heal within 6 to 8 weeks with nonoperative measures, such as immobilization or reduction in strenuous activity. Impaired BLT healing, however, is frequently encountered in both inpatient and outpatient situations. Impaired BLT healing is associated with risk factors, such as extreme of age, estrogen deficiency, smoking, osteoporosis, diabetes mellitus, alcohol abuse, obesity, noncompliance, chronic site infection, deformity, and neuropathy. Impairment of BLT healing can have devastating consequences to the patient and may lead to injury-related morbidity and mortality. Poor fifth metatarsal healing and Charcot neuropathic osteoarthropathy (CN) are both clinically challenging conditions that result from impaired BLT healing. Arthrodesis is a common procedure used to resolve many foot and ankle conditions like CN. Complications with this procedure, however, are frequent in populations with comorbidities and risk factors. The pathogenesis, etiology, and current treatment challenges for fifth metatarsal and CN are reviewed.

Fifth Metatarsal Fractures: Epidemiology, Pathogenesis, and Diagnosis

Stress and damage induced by direct and indirect injuries to the bone are typically healed by the natural bone remodeling process. Direct damage, such as high-impact trauma, including motor vehicle accidents or heavy falling objects, can apply a direct force and lead to metatarsal fractures at any location.[39] In contrast, indirect forces applying torque to the foot can result in fractures of the metatarsal shafts.[40] Repetitive stress or chronic damage of a metatarsal can overwhelm the normal remodeling process and weaken spots in the bone, leading to the development of stress fractures. Metatarsal fractures account for 35% of all foot fractures and approximately 25% result from stress fractures of the fifth metatarsal.[41-43] Unlike normal fractures, stress fractures do not heal by callus formation; instead, they undergo direct remodeling.[44,45] Direct remodeling to heal stress fractures is slow and often stress fractures progress to complete fractures, which resist healing and often lead to nonunion.[44,45] Patients with metatarsal fractures typically show signs of antalgic gait, dorsal edema, and ecchymosis. Clinical, neurovascular, physical, and radiographic evaluations are used to diagnose metatarsal fractures.[46]

Fifth Metatarsal Fractures: Anatomic Considerations

Of the metatarsals, fifth metatarsal fractures are the most common. They account for 68% of metatarsal fractures in populations between 20 and 50 years old.[47,48] The fifth metatarsal consists of a base, neck, head, the tuberosity, and the diaphysis (shaft). The lateral band of plantar fascia, the peroneus brevis tendon, and the peroneus teritus tendon are all soft tissues associated with the fifth metatarsal.[49,50] The osteology of the fifth metatarsal is curved and the dorsal-plantar cortex is thinner than the medial-lateral cortex. Blood supply around the fifth metatarsal varies. The tuberosity's blood supply comes from multiple metaphyseal vessels and multiple branches of the nutrient artery. The proximal diaphysis, however, receives its blood supply solely from the nutrient artery.[51,52] Fracture in the proximal diaphysis is more likely to disrupt the blood supply and contributes to high rates of nonunion, delayed union, or refracture.[53] Proximal fifth metatarsal fractures are sometimes classified into 3 anatomic zones. Zone I is the most proximal and includes the tuberosity. Zone II is the metadiaphyseal junction and includes the Jones fracture region. Zone III occurs at the proximal diaphysis. Fractures occurring in zone I and zone II usually occur from direct and indirect acute damage whereas fractures in zone III result from pathologic stress.[54]

Fifth Metatarsal Fractures: Treatment and Challenges

For treatment and prognoses reasons, fractures in the fifth metatarsal are classified into types I, II, and III.[50] Type I fractures involve the tip of tuberosity and have been associated with sport-related injuries. These tuberosity avulsion fractures occur during inversions of the foot and ankle while they are in plantar flexion. Studies have shown that both the lateral band of plantar fascia and the peroneus brevis are involved.[39,55] Type I injuries are usually completely healed within 6 to 8 weeks if the avulsion fracture is nondisplaced. Conservative treatment includes rest, ice, elevation above heart level, and often a soft Jones dressing with stiff-soled shoe, non–weight-bearing short leg cast, or removable controlled ankle motion walker. Complications from type I fractures are unusual, although Bigsby and colleagues[56] recently demonstrated in a prospective study that 25% of patients have pain a year after the injury. This discomfort is typically correlated with displaced fractures that may lead to nonunion. If a nonunion persists, some clinicians use pulsed electromagnetic field therapy or external bone stimulators to promote healing. Pulsed electromagnetic field therapy has been effectively used in the management of delayed unions and nonunions of type I fractures whereas little research has been conducted on the efficacy of other bone stimulators.[40,56,57]

In type I fractures, surgical intervention is necessary if displacement is greater than 3 mm, a step-off of more than 1 mm to 2 mm on the articular surface with the cuboid, 30% of the metatarsal cuboid joint articulation is involved, or if callus formation is not evident by the eighth week after radiographic examination.[39,58,59] Surgical interventions for fifth metatarsal fractures vary but include screw fixation, tension banding, and percutaneous pinning.[42,55,60-66] In 1 study, the effectiveness of percutaneous biocortical screw fixation for displaced intra-articular zone I proximal fifth metatarsals was studied.[64] The data demonstrated that percutaneous biocortical screw fixation effectively decreased preoperative displacement and allowed for complete healing within 4 to 6 weeks. Biocortical fixation was suggested as superior to intramedullary fixation because it disperses the load over a greater cortex surface area and offers greater stability.

Type II injuries occur within the junction of the metaphysis and diaphysis and generally result from an acute sports injury.[67] Unlike type I injuries, type II injuries are not caused by inversion. These fractures are thought to develop when a significant adduction force is applied to the forefoot while the ankle is in plantar flexion.[59] Stress fractures can also develop in this area and need to be successfully distinguished from an acute injury to develop a proper treatment plan for the patient. Clinical presentation, patient history, and radiographic findings need to be carefully examined to differentiate between acute and stress fractures. Initial treatment requires immobilization in a posterior splint, strict non–weight bearing, icing, and elevation of the limb. For most nondisplaced acute fractures, conservative treatment is recommended.[39,59,67]

Acute type II diaphyseal fractures, however, pose several challenges for successful healing. Because it is difficult to distinguish between acute and stress fractures, incorrect diagnosis often leads to improper treatment and results in a high incidence of nonunion. Therefore, it is important to gain a thorough patient history and carefully examine all radiographs to properly diagnose the patient. Also, treatment of acute diaphyseal fractures requires casting and strict non–weight bearing for long periods of time so many patients are noncompliant. Even with proper diagnosis and treatment, many acute diaphyseal fractures result in nonunion or refracture.[59] In a study of basketball players carefully diagnosed with acute proximal diaphysis injury, 50% percent were found unhealed after 12 weeks of conservative treatment.[68] Impaired vascular supply and premature weight bearing are thought to cause poor healing in these injuries.[52,53,67] A 2005 study compared conservative and surgical treatment of these fractures.[69] In this study, approximately 50% of the patients were treated with intramedullary screw fixation followed by immobilization for a period of 2 weeks. The remaining 50% of the patients were immobilized in a non–weight bearing, short leg cast for 8 weeks, followed by a walking cast, until there was radiographic and clinical evidence on fracture union; 44% of the conservatively treated group were found to have a visible symptomatic fracture 26 weeks postfracture whereas only 5% of the surgically treated group did. Two other articles, which reviewed 32 studies, showed that surgical intervention generally reduced the risk of nonunion.[70,71] As a result of these challenges, early surgical fixation and prolonged use of a customized weight-bearing orthosis are reasonable options for treatments.[67,72]

Type III injuries include stress fractures of the fifth metatarsal and result from chronic and repetitive microtrauma. Type III fractures occur less frequently then type I and II fractures; however, they have a much higher propensity to develop into a delayed union, nonunion, or refracture.[59,73] Radiographically they are distinct from acute fractures and have been classified by Torg based on severity.[74] An early stress fracture displays cortical thickening (Torg I) whereas older stress fractures have a thicker fracture line (Torg II) or absence of the medullary canal (Torg III). Most type III injuries require surgical fixation (Torg II and III) instead of conservative treatment (Torg I).[75] Conservative treatment is advised only for patients with early stress fractures who would like to avoid surgery and do not mind long-term immobilization. Surgical fixation, bone stimulators, bone grafts, and other therapies have been used to manage problematic stress fractures and are similar to the options already discussed for acute metatarsal injuries. Surgical treatment of these fractures has similar challenges and healing outcomes as described for type II metatarsal fractures. Operative treatment still results, however, in prolonged immobilization time.[42,54,63–65] Current research is focused on improving the surgical methods to reduce the time a patient is prohibited from activities. One study using teriparatide, a Food and Drug Administration–approved bone stimulator for osteoporosis treatment, focused on improving healing outcomes without surgical intervention.[42] Improvement was seen in 2 patients with metatarsal stress fracture healing after treatment with teriparatide, vitamin D_3, and calcium citrate. The scope of this study was limited, however, and future studies are warranted. A future study aims to test the efficacy of adding bone marrow stem cells to the surgical site to promote better healing outcomes for metatarsal stress fractures.[65] Continued research on these specific injuries is warranted and could result in improved healing success in patients with type III fractures as well as those suffering from type I and II fractures.

Charcot Neuropathic Osteoarthropathy: Epidemiology, Pathogenesis, and Diagnosis

CN, commonly known as Charcot foot, is a condition where acute localized inflammation affects the bones, joints, and soft tissues of the foot and ankle. CN results from various peripheral neuropathies but is commonly associated with diabetic neuropathy. The precise incidence of CN is unclear but it was recently estimated to effect 0.08% to 0.13% of the population but has a higher incidence in the diabetic community (7.5%–9%).[76–78] CN can be classified in terms of clinical stage, anatomic localization, and stage of natural history, which have been described extensively in the literature.[78–81] Proper and prompt diagnosis of CN is important to minimize the risk of osteophyte development, ulceration, infection, deformity, and amputation. Recent studies demonstrate that plain radiographs are insufficient at diagnosing Charcot foot injuries.[9,82,83] Many studies have shown that advanced imaging, such as MRIs, are better at properly diagnosing CN.[9,83–90]

CN's cause is thought to be multifactorial resulting from several components, such as diabetes, sensory-motor neuropathy, or metabolic abnormalities of the bone. These components contribute to unresolved acute inflammation in a specific ankle or foot region, which inflicts varying degrees of bone damage, subluxation, dislocation, and deformity. Midfoot collapse, commonly known as rocker-bottom foot, is a classic deformity associated with CN. The pathogenesis or process by which CN progresses is not well understood; however, 2 theories have been described.[78] The neurovascular theory states that an autonomic stimulated vascular reflex causes hyperemia and increased bone resorption, which leads to joint destruction and trauma. The neurotraumatic theory suggests that CN results from peripheral neuropathy, which causes sensory loss in the feet. As a result, repetitive strain, pain, and overload are unrecognized in the insensate region, which eventually leads to unknown trauma or injury that triggers the development of CN.[78,91–94]

Charcot Neuropathic Osteoarthropathy: Anatomic Considerations

CN's classification systems have varied over the years; for simplicity, this review uses the classic model to describe the stages of this condition. Stage I is the acute phase and is characterized by fragmentation. The midfoot is usually affected and is characterized by swelling and warmth. Some radiographs display osteopenia, periarticular fragmentation, and subluxation of joints but most seem typically normal. The acute stage is often misdiagnosed as gout, deep vein thrombosis, or soft tissue injury and as a result the disease can progress to stage II or stage III.[95–98] Stage II represents the reparative phase where edema and warmth decrease, bone absorption occurs, and bone formation occur. Stage III is known as the chronic or inactive stage.[78–80,99]

Many of the acute signs, such as warmth and redness, disappear, but stable deformities may develop in the third stage.[78–80,99] Common deformities to develop include collapse of the plantar arch in the midfoot or a prominent medial aspect of the midfoot. These deformities often result in formation of abnormally high-pressure areas on the foot that become particularly prone to ulceration.[78–80,99]

Charcot Neuropathic Osteoarthropathy: Treatment and Challenges

It is of utmost importance that CN be properly diagnosed and treated during the acute stage to prevent further progression of the condition. Conservative treatment is typical in stage I and includes immobilization with a nonremovable device, such as a total contact cast, with instructions to be non–weight bearing. Literature exists that suggests that weight bearing while immobilized does not negatively affect the resolution of acute CN.[9,82,83,89,98,100,101] The duration of immobilization is dependent on the extremity and radiographic evidence of ossification at the site but on average it can range between 8 and 52 weeks.[77,82,84,87,89,95,98] Conservative treatment, however, has its challenges. Prolonged casting and immobilization can lead to complications, such as ulceration, and patient compliance during prolonged immobilization periods is not easy to guarantee.[97,101–104] Other orthotic devices are available (removable walking boots and patellar tendon brace) that help increase patient compliance although studies indicate that use of the orthotic devices increases the length of time patients are immobile.[98,105,106] Surgical intervention during this acute stage has some major risks for wound healing complications and infection.[87,98,99,103,107,108] Additionally, bone quality is a main concern because CN is characterized by the pathogenic process of osteoclastic resorption and fragmentation. The bone quality is feared to be suboptimal for proper fixation, which could lead to hardware failure, pseudoarthritis, delayed union, or nonunions.[98,99,108] Therefore, surgery in the acute phase of CN is restricted to patients with severe dislocation or instability, failure of conservative treatment, poor vascular supply near the affected limb, patients with comorbidities, or evidence of an anatomic location breakdown. Early surgical intervention during acute CN in diabetic patients was found effective at increasing arthrodesis without complications.[108] Stage II is considered a better time for surgical intervention. Surgical intervention is typically completed with an open reduction and internal fixation.[82] If the process has reached the stage III, arthrodesis is typically more difficult to achieve because an ostectomy needs to be conducted and may result in ulcerations.[82,97,102,109]

Surgical intervention for CN includes nonlocking and locking plate and screw fixation, intramedullary screw or nail fixation, external fixation, internal fixation, or a combination of these methods.[110–112] Surgical method choice is typically dependent on bone quality. If bone quality is poor, internal fixation may use a superconstruct[113,114] that connects affected joints to nonaffected joints to gain stability. This method requires large incisions, however, which increase the risk of infection, soft tissue complications, and disruption to the osseous vascular supply.[110] Intramedullary screw and nail fixation require a smaller open approach and thus limit the risks associated with a large incision. Intramedullary fixation also gives clinicians the ability to correct and realign deformed bone with use of guide wires, but complications resulting from hardware failure or migration can occur.[5,110,113–119] External fixation is used with or without internal fixation if a patient is suffering from severe deformity or instability. Most external devices use tensioned wires to stabilize multiple planes and promote interfragmentary compression to prevent implant loosing, neutralize stress placed on the foot, and assist in deformity correction.[112,120,121] Complications resulting from external fixation are more common in diabetic patients and include pin loosening, pin breakage, pin failure, stress fractures, osteomyelitis, and pin tract infections.[122]

If surgical correction requires arthrodesis, the use of bone graft and/or adjuvants may be necessary. Autogenic bone is typically preferred but allogenic, synthetic, or combinatorial bone graft substitutes can be used. Autogenic bone graft is typically harvested from the iliac crest, distal tibia, or fibula and is used to fill osseous voids.[123–126] Disadvantages of autogenic bone use are donor site morbidity, pain, and availability.[123] Allogenic grafts avoid the disadvantages associated with autogenic bones and reduce the operating time needed to obtain the bone. Other bone graft substitutes, such as demineralized bone matrix, calcium sulfates, and hydroxyapatites are also readily available as alternatives to allogenic grafts. Incorporating orthobiologics, such as BMP, bone marrow aspirate, or platelet-rich plasma, into the wound or osseous region can enhance healing.[82,127,128] In a recent study, patients at high risk for surgical failure (those who are immunodeficient or have multiple comorbidities or recurrent infections) underwent CN surgery for deformity correction using allogenic bone graft supplemented with platelet-rich plasma.[129] Arthrodesis was achieved in 90% of the patients and that were also infection-free at 26 months. Similar favorable outcomes have been achieved with adjunctive treatments, such as bisphosphonates,[106] intranasal calcitonin,[130] and bone stimulation.[57]

Because CN can be challenging to diagnosis and treat, it is recommended that advanced imaging be conducted on any patient with peripheral neuropathy, pain, and swelling to rule out acute CN. Immobilization seems the preferred treatment of acute-stage CN even though some evidence suggest surgery at this stage can improve outcomes. When surgical intervention is necessary, use of orthobiologics or adjuvants seems to increase positive healing outcomes.

Arthrodesis of the Foot and Ankle

Fusion of the foot or ankle is typically used as an end-stage procedure to salvage the limb. Patients with certain risk factors, such as smoking, diabetes, alcohol abuse, obesity, or genetic disorders, are at greater risk for complications associated with fusion. Surgical techniques to promote fusion are numerous and include use of internal and external fixation. Examples of these methods are discussed previously regarding treating stage II and III Charcot foot. Complications are common with arthrodesis and include hardware failure, pin migration, infection, delayed union, nonunion, stress fractures, and cortical hypertrophy. Biological augmentation with osteoconductive or osteoinductive reagents have been the focus of research to increase fusion success. Some studies show promising results with use of osteobiologics, such as recombinant human BMP-2 to promote arthrodesis,[23,131,132] although others note complications, such as heterotopic ossification.[23,133,134] For an extensive review of the challenges involved in arthrodesis, see Rabinovich and colleagues[23] and Slater and colleagues[135] on complex ankle arthrodesis.

BIOLOGY OF LIGAMENT AND TENDON HEALING
Ligament and Tendon Healing

Tendon and ligament ruptures and tears are common injuries. Acute tendon and ligament injuries are often caused by extrinsic traumatic injuries.[136] Rapid acceleration-deceleration movements have been associated, however, with acute sports-related tendon injuries.[137] Chronic degenerative changes in tendons and ligaments also can lead to susceptibility for rupture or tear.[138] Possible mechanisms leading to chronic degenerative changes in tendon include damage from reactive oxygen species produced in conjunction with load-induced ischemia-reperfusion,[139] strain-induced cyclooxygenase expression leading to prostaglandin E_2 synthesis, inflammation, and matrix metalloproteinase synthesis and accumulated small partial tears that would weaken the overall tensile strength of the tendon.[140–143] Use of fluoroquinolone antibiotics, such as ciprofloxacin, also has been associated with increased risk of tendon rupture.[144,145] Cell-based studies have shown that ciprofloxacin can induce IL-1ß expression that could possible trigger inflammation-related tendon damage,[146] although others have suggested that IL-1ß may not be involved in tendinopathy.[147]

Treating tendon and ligament injuries is complicated by an incomplete understanding of how tendons and ligaments heal. For instance, there is significant variation in the ability of some ligaments to heal because knee medial collateral ligament injuries are often managed nonsurgically during healing whereas knee anterior cruciate ligament injuries generally undergo surgical repair.[148–150] The location of the injury may also affect treatment and outcomes, such as management of adhesion formation, in injuries involving the tendon sheath or injuries involving the muscle-tendon (myotendinous) junction or the bone-tendon interface (enthesis).

Unlike bone, tendons and ligaments do not heal by tissue regeneration but rather through a typical wound healing process in which the defect is filled with fibrous tissue. Complete or partial disruption of the tendon or ligament leads to a predictable healing pathway that includes an early phase, reparative phase, and a remodeling phase that increases repaired tendon tensile properties. The early phase consists of hematoma formation, inflammation, and initiation of cell proliferation at the injury site. During the reparative phase, proliferating tenocytes from the tendon and epitenon and proliferating cells from surrounding tissues, for example, the tendon sheath, localize at the injury site and begin to heal the rupture by formation of fibrous tissue that contains a high proportion of type III collagen. This reparative phase can last for weeks during which time the healing tendon remains mechanically weak and subject to reinjury. During the remodeling phase, the fibrous repair tissue becomes less cellular, glycosaminoglycan concentrations decrease, and the proportion of type I collagen increases. Eventually the collagen fibers and tenocytes align with the direction of stress to increase the repaired tendon tensile strength. The remodeling phase can last several months. Factors that mediate inflammation, angiogenesis, cell proliferation, and extracellular matrix remodeling seem to be involved in the different phases of healing based on gene expression studies. The mechanisms that coordinate these gene expression events, however, and the necessity of each factor in tendon healing are not well understood.

Recent studies have cataloged patterns of gene expression after tendon or ligament injuries. Using a mouse flexor tendon defect model, Juneja and colleagues[151] found a rapid increase in in type III collagen expression that peaked between 2 and 3 weeks after surgery. Expression of anti-inflammatory TGF-ß3 increased approximately 6-fold between 7 and 14 days after fracture, which coincides with the transition from the early to reparative phase of healing. Manning and colleagues[152] found that type III and type I collagen expression was reduced more than 10-fold immediately after canine flexor tendon transection and repair compared with normal tendon, whereas inflammatory-related gene expression (IL-1ß and cyclooxygenase-2) was elevated. Manning and colleagues also observed that after 9 days, type III collagen gene expression had increased suggesting initiation of the reparative phase. More recent gene expression studies have been conducted using human tendon samples collected during surgery. Using microarrays, Brophy and colleagues analyzed gene expression between anterior-cruciate ligaments that had been torn less than 3 months (acute), between 3 and 12 months (intermediate), or greater than 12 months (chronic).[153] Ends of the torn ligaments were collected during surgical repair and so no intact specimens were available for comparison. Still, the analysis found that genes involved in extracellular matrix reorganization were expressed in the acute samples, whereas the chronic samples showed reductions in collagen gene expression and an interesting greater than 30-fold decline in periostin expression. Chaudhury and colleagues[154] compared rotator cuff tendons that had been symptomatic for at least 1 year with small (<3 cm) and large (>3 cm) tears to control rotator cuff tendons using microarrays. The results confirmed many previous studies, such as significant changes in extracellular matrix remodeling gene expression. Perhaps more important, analysis of the microarray data showed clear demarcations in gene expression patterns between the 3 different groups, indicating significant differences in the injury response between small and large tears.

The Tendon Sheath and Adhesions

A complication associated with tendon injuries is formation of adhesions between the tendon and the surrounding sheath or other tissues that limits range of motion.[155,156] Cellular continuity between the tendon and surrounding tissue often occurs after injury as cells proliferate from the tendon and surrounding tissue to form the initial fibrous repair tissue. These cellular continuities must be resolved, however, to allow the tendon to move freely and without limiting the range of motion. Nominally, these cellular continuities are resolved during healing and can be aided by early movement of the healing tendon and by nonsteroidal anti-inflammatory drug treatment.[157,158] Failure to resolve the cellular continuities seems to lead to adhesion formation. Given the nature of the adhesions, the pathologic mechanism leading to adhesion formation could be failure to slow cell proliferation during the repair phase, failure to stop production of predominant type III collagen fibrous tissue, failure to produce sufficient levels of extracellular matrix remodeling enzymes, or a combination of these processes.[151] Additional research is needed to understand the etiology of adhesion formation and for improving methods to prevent adhesion formation.

Healing at the Enthesis and Myotendinous Junction

Tendons and ligaments are connected to bone through a specialized fibrocartilage and calcified fibrocartilage structure called the enthesis.[159–162] Tendons connect to muscle at myotendinous junctions in which the tendon collagen fibrils interact with the sarcolemma of the muscle to allow force transmission.[163] Despite the efficiency with which mechanical forces are transmitted through the enthesis and myotendinous junction, these junctions are mechanical weak points and sites of degenerative changes. Ruptures at myotendinous junctions seem to heal well and are often treated nonsurgically.[164] In contrast, healing of ruptured entheses is more problematic and typically the normal structure of the enthesis is not rejuvenated. Instead, in the repaired tendon-bone junction, the tendon and bone are joined by fibrocartilage.[165,166]

Current Research Areas

There is as yet no gold standard animal model for studying tendon repair, which makes comparison of gene expression and other data between models and species difficult. Complete and partial transection of the mouse Achilles tendon may be the best model to study the basic molecular and cellular events associated with tendon healing. The mouse Achilles tendon model allows for partial or complete transection for no or simple suture repair as well as testing of biomaterials and grafts. The mouse allows for use of genetically modified animals to directly assess gene functions on tendon healing, and healing can be measured using molecular, histologic, and mechanical methods.[167–173] Any conclusion drawn from mouse Achilles tendon studies, however, needs to be confirmed using clinical samples because there are clear differences in healing potentials between different tendons and species.

Research to improve tendon and ligament healing, improve healing at the enthesis or myotendinous junction, and prevents or minimizes adhesions is ongoing.[136,174,175] Efforts are focused on manipulating inflammation,[158,176–180] using growth factors to control cell fates,[33,181] altering extracellular matrix reorganization,[182,183] and development of grafting materials.[184] Another concept being explored is to recreate a healing environment that recapitulates that which occurs during fetal development to promote scarless wound healing.[185]

SUMMARY

Multiple factors, such as genetic predisposition, comorbidities, anatomy, proper and prompt diagnosis, treatment type (conservative or surgical), and patient compliance, all contribute to the challenges associated with effectively treating fifth metatarsal injury, CN, and arthrodesis. Even though these conditions have been extensively studied, successfully healing these conditions is still difficult. Research suggests that effective treatment begins with rapid and accurate diagnosis of the condition, which is best completed using advancing imaging, such as MRI. The stage of the condition, patient risk factors, and comorbidities dictate whether conservative treatment or surgical intervention is necessary. Conservative treatment often leads to refracture, nonunion, or secondary complications like ulceration or infection. Failed conservative treatment eventually leads to surgical intervention. Surgical intervention can include internal fixation, external fixation, bone grafts, orthobiologics, adjuvants, or a combination of these methods, each of which has its drawbacks, including pin migration, heterotopic ossification, or hardware failure. Despite these disadvantages, conservative and surgical treatment can be successful. Additional randomized controlled trials, however, applying new or improved methods needs to be conducted to justify their use on BLT-related injuries in the future.

REFERENCES

1. De Boer AS, Schepers T, Panneman MJ, et al. Health care consumption and costs due to foot and ankle injuries in the Netherlands, 1986-2010. BMC Musculoskelet Disord 2014;15:128.
2. Einhorn TA, Gerstenfeld LC. Fracture healing: mechanisms and interventions. Nat Rev Rheumatol 2015;11(1):45–54.
3. Gomez-Barrena E, Rosset P, Lozano D, et al. Bone fracture healing: cell therapy in delayed unions and nonunions. Bone 2015;70:93–101.
4. Begkas D, Katsenis D, Pastroudis A. Management of aseptic non-unions of the distal third of the tibial diaphysis using static interlocking intramedullary nailing. Med Glas (Zenica) 2014;11(1):159–64.
5. Assal M, Stern R. Realignment and extended fusion with use of a medial column screw for midfoot deformities secondary to diabetic neuropathy. J Bone Joint Surg Am 2009;91(4):812–20.
6. Pacicca DM, Patel N, Lee C, et al. Expression of angiogenic factors during distraction osteogenesis. Bone 2003;33(6):889–98.
7. Phillips AM. Overview of the fracture healing cascade. Injury 2005;36(Suppl 3): S5–7.
8. Stoffel K, Engler H, Kuster M, et al. Changes in biochemical markers after lower limb fractures. Clin Chem 2007;53(1):131–4.

9. Chantelau EA, Grutzner G. Is the Eichenholtz classification still valid for the diabetic Charcot foot? Swiss Med Wkly 2014;144:w13948.
10. Dennis SC, Berkland CJ, Bonewald LF, et al. Endochondral ossification for enhancing bone regeneration: converging native extracellular matrix biomaterials and developmental engineering in vivo. Tissue Eng Part B Rev 2015; 21(3):247–66.
11. Lin HN, Cottrell J, O'Connor JP. Variation in lipid mediator and cytokine levels during mouse femur fracture healing. J Orthop Res 2016. [Epub ahead of print].
12. Schlundt C, El Khassawna T, Serra A, et al. Macrophages in bone fracture healing: Their essential role in endochondral ossification. Bone 2015. [Epub ahead of print].
13. Colnot C. Skeletal cell fate decisions within periosteum and bone marrow during bone regeneration. J Bone Miner Res 2009;24(2):274–82.
14. Vortkamp A, Pathi S, Peretti GM, et al. Recapitulation of signals regulating embryonic bone formation during postnatal growth and in fracture repair. Mech Dev 1998;71(1–2):65–76.
15. Mackie EJ, Ahmed YA, Tatarczuch L, et al. Endochondral ossification: how cartilage is converted into bone in the developing skeleton. Int J Biochem Cell Biol 2008;40(1):46–62.
16. Marsell R, Einhorn TA. The biology of fracture healing. Injury 2011;42(6):551–5.
17. Sfeir C, Ho L, Doll BA, et al. Fracture repair. In: Lieberman JR, Friedlaender GE, editors. Bone regeneration and repair. Totowa (NJ): Humana Press Inc.; 2005. p. 21–44.
18. Reinholt FP, Hultenby K, Oldberg A, et al. Osteopontin–a possible anchor of osteoclasts to bone. Proc Natl Acad Sci U S A 1990;87(12):4473–5.
19. Clarke B. Normal bone anatomy and physiology. Clin J Am Soc Nephrol 2008; 3(Suppl 3):S131–9.
20. Hadjidakis DJ, Androulakis II. Bone remodeling. Ann N Y Acad Sci 2006;1092: 385–96.
21. Kalfas IH. Principles of bone healing. Neurosurg Focus 2001;10(4):E1.
22. Gougoulias N, Lampridis V. Midfoot arthrodesis. Foot Ankle Surg 2016;22(1): 17–25.
23. Rabinovich RV, Haleem AM, Rozbruch SR. Complex ankle arthrodesis: Review of the literature. World J Orthop 2015;6(8):602–13.
24. Hardy MA, Logan DB. Principles of arthrodesis and advances in fixation for the adult acquired flatfoot. Clin Podiatr Med Surg 2007;24(4):789–813, x.
25. Saltzman CL, Kadoko RG, Suh JS. Treatment of isolated ankle osteoarthritis with arthrodesis or the total ankle replacement: a comparison of early outcomes. Clin Orthop Surg 2010;2(1):1–7.
26. Terrell RD, Montgomery SR, Pannell WC, et al. Comparison of practice patterns in total ankle replacement and ankle fusion in the United States. Foot Ankle Int 2013;34(11):1486–92.
27. Xiaobing Y, Dewei Z, Weiming W. Evaluation of clinical effect of ankle arthrodesis and total ankle arthroplasty for end-stage ankle arthritis. Clin Res Foot Ankle 2014;2(129). p. 1–3.
28. Hayden RJ, Jebson PJ. Wrist arthrodesis. Hand Clin 2005;21(4):631–40.
29. Dux K, Edgar S, Blume P. A guide to the triple arthrodesis for hindfoot deformities. Podiatry Today 2012;25. HMP Communications, LLC.
30. Schuh R, Salzberger F, Wanivenhaus AH, et al. Kinematic changes in patients with double arthrodesis of the hindfoot for realignment of planovalgus deformity. J Orthop Res 2013;31(4):517–24.

31. Capobianco R, Cher D, Group SS. Safety and effectiveness of minimally invasive sacroiliac joint fusion in women with persistent post-partum posterior pelvic girdle pain: 12-month outcomes from a prospective, multi-center trial. Springerplus 2015;4:570.

32. Rutherford EE, Tarplett LJ, Davies EM, et al. Lumbar spine fusion and stabilization: hardware, techniques, and imaging appearances. Radiographics 2007; 27(6):1737–49.

33. Akyol E, Hindocha S, Khan WS. Use of stem cells and growth factors in rotator cuff tendon repair. Curr Stem Cel Res Ther 2014;10(1):5–10.

34. Weiss HR, Goodall D. Rate of complications in scoliosis surgery - a systematic review of the Pub Med literature. Scoliosis 2008;3:9.

35. Kovack TJ, Jacob PB, Mighell MA. Elbow arthrodesis: a novel technique and review of the literature. Orthopedics 2014;37(5):313–9.

36. Schafroth MU, Blokzijl RJ, Haverkamp D, et al. The long-term fate of the hip arthrodesis: does it remain a valid procedure for selected cases in the 21st century? Int Orthop 2010;34(6):805–10.

37. Bonasia DE, Dettoni F, Femino JE, et al. Total ankle replacement: why, when and how? Iowa Orthop J 2010;30:119–30.

38. AOFAS. Position Statement: the use of total ankle replacement for the treatment of arthritic conditions of the ankle. American Orthopaedic Foot & Ankle Society, Rosemont, IL; 2014.

39. Lawrence SJ, Botte MJ. Jones' fractures and related fractures of the proximal fifth metatarsal. Foot Ankle 1993;14(6):358–65.

40. Richli WR, Rosenthal DI. Avulsion fracture of the fifth metatarsal: experimental study of pathomechanics. AJR Am J Roentgenol 1984;143(4):889–91.

41. Burge R, Dawson-Hughes B, Solomon DH, et al. Incidence and economic burden of osteoporosis-related fractures in the United States, 2005-2025. J Bone Miner Res 2007;22(3):465–75.

42. Raghavan P, Christofides E. Role of teriparatide in accelerating metatarsal stress fracture healing: a case series and review of literature. Clin Med Insights Endocrinol Diabetes 2012;5:39–45.

43. Urteaga AJ, Lynch M. Fractures of the central metatarsals. Clin Podiatr Med Surg 1995;12(4):759–72.

44. Fazzalari NL. Bone fracture and bone fracture repair. Osteoporos Int 2011;22(6): 2003–6.

45. Kidd LJ, Stephens AS, Kuliwaba JS, et al. Temporal pattern of gene expression and histology of stress fracture healing. Bone 2010;46(2):369–78.

46. Hatch RL, Alsobrook JA, Clugston JR. Diagnosis and management of metatarsal fractures. Am Fam Physician 2007;76(6):817–26.

47. Petrisor BA, Ekrol I, Court-Brown C. The epidemiology of metatarsal fractures. Foot Ankle Int 2006;27(3):172–4.

48. Petrisor BA, Poolman R, Koval K, et al. Management of displaced ankle fractures. J Orthop Trauma 2006;20(7):515–8.

49. Rammelt S, Heineck J, Zwipp H. Metatarsal fractures. Injury 2004;35(Suppl 2): SB77–86.

50. Strayer SM, Reece SG, Petrizzi MJ. Fractures of the proximal fifth metatarsal. Am Fam Physician 1999;59(9):2516–22.

51. Shereff MJ, Sobel MA, Kummer FJ. The stability of fixation of first metatarsal osteotomies. Foot Ankle 1991;11(4):208–11.

52. Shereff MJ, Yang QM, Kummer FJ, et al. Vascular anatomy of the fifth metatarsal. Foot Ankle 1991;11(6):350–3.

53. Smith JW, Arnoczky SP, Hersh A. The intraosseous blood supply of the fifth metatarsal: implications for proximal fracture healing. Foot Ankle 1992;13(3): 143–52.
54. Tahririan MA, Momeni A, Moayednia A, et al. Designing a prognostic scoring system for predicting the outcomes of proximal fifth metatarsal fractures at 20 weeks. Iran J Med Sci 2015;40(2):104–9.
55. Theodorou DJ, Theodorou SJ, Kakitsubata Y, et al. Fractures of proximal portion of fifth metatarsal bone: anatomic and imaging evidence of a pathogenesis of avulsion of the plantar aponeurosis and the short peroneal muscle tendon. Radiology 2003;226(3):857–65.
56. Bigsby E, Halliday R, Middleton RG, et al. Functional outcome of fifth metatarsal fractures. Injury 2014;45(12):2009–12.
57. Hanft JR, Goggin JP, Landsman A, et al. The role of combined magnetic field bone growth stimulation as an adjunct in the treatment of neuroarthropathy/ Charcot joint: an expanded pilot study. J Foot Ankle Surg 1998;37(6):510–5 [discussion: 550–1].
58. Mehlhorn AT, Zwingmann J, Hirschmuller A, et al. Radiographic classification for fractures of the fifth metatarsal base. Skeletal Radiol 2014;43(4):467–74.
59. Quill GE Jr. Fractures of the proximal fifth metatarsal. Orthop Clin North Am 1995;26(2):353–61.
60. Glasgow MT, Naranja RJ Jr, Glasgow SG, et al. Analysis of failed surgical management of fractures of the base of the fifth metatarsal distal to the tuberosity: the Jones fracture. Foot Ankle Int 1996;17(8):449–57.
61. Husain ZS, DeFronzo DJ. Relative stability of tension band versus two-cortex screw fixation for treating fifth metatarsal base avulsion fractures. J Foot Ankle Surg 2000;39(2):89–95.
62. Husain ZS, DeFronzo DJ. A comparison of bicortical and intramedullary screw fixations of Jones' fractures. J Foot Ankle Surg 2002;41(3):146–53.
63. Lui TH. Lateral foot pain following open reduction and internal fixation of the fracture of the fifth metatarsal tubercle: treated by arthroscopic arthrolysis and endoscopic tenolysis. BMJ Case Rep 2014;1–4.
64. Mahajan V, Chung HW, Suh JS. Fractures of the proximal fifth metatarsal: percutaneous bicortical fixation. Clin Orthop Surg 2011;3(2):140–6.
65. Weel H, Mallee WH, van Dijk CN, et al. The effect of concentrated bone marrow aspirate in operative treatment of fifth metatarsal stress fractures; a double-blind randomized controlled trial. BMC Musculoskelet Disord 2015;16:211.
66. Wright RW, Fischer DA, Shively RA, et al. Refracture of proximal fifth metatarsal (Jones) fracture after intramedullary screw fixation in athletes. Am J Sports Med 2000;28(5):732–6.
67. Nunley JA. Fractures of the base of the fifth metatarsal: the Jones fracture. Orthop Clin North Am 2001;32(1):171–80.
68. Fernandez Fairen M, Guillen J, Busto JM, et al. Fractures of the fifth metatarsal in basketball players. Knee Surg Sports Traumatol Arthrosc 1999;7(6):373–7.
69. Mologne TS, Lundeen JM, Clapper MF, et al. Early screw fixation versus casting in the treatment of acute Jones fractures. Am J Sports Med 2005;33(7):970–5.
70. Roche AJ, Calder JD. Treatment and return to sport following a Jones fracture of the fifth metatarsal: a systematic review. Knee Surg Sports Traumatol Arthrosc 2013;21(6):1307–15.
71. Yates J, Feeley I, Sasikumar S, et al. Jones fracture of the fifth metatarsal: Is operative intervention justified? A systematic review of the literature and meta-analysis of results. Foot (Edinb) 2015;25(4):251–7.

72. Dameron TB Jr. Fractures and anatomical variations of the proximal portion of the fifth metatarsal. J Bone Joint Surg Am 1975;57(6):788–92.
73. DeLee JC, Evans JP, Julian J. Stress fracture of the fifth metatarsal. Am J Sports Med 1983;11(5):349–53.
74. Torg JS, Balduini FC, Zelko RR, et al. Fractures of the base of the fifth metatarsal distal to the tuberosity. Classification and guidelines for non-surgical and surgical management. J Bone Joint Surg Am 1984;66(2):209–14.
75. Zwitser EW, Breederveld RS. Fractures of the fifth metatarsal; diagnosis and treatment. Injury 2010;41(6):555–62.
76. Klenerman L. The Charcot joint in diabetes. Diabet Med 1996;13(Suppl 1): S52–4.
77. Sinha S, Munichoodappa CS, Kozak GP. Neuro-arthropathy (Charcot joints) in diabetes mellitus (clinical study of 101 cases). Medicine (Baltimore) 1972; 51(3):191–210.
78. van der Ven A, Chapman CB, Bowker JH. Charcot neuroarthropathy of the foot and ankle. J Am Acad Orthop Surg 2009;17(9):562–71.
79. Gouveri E, Papanas N. Charcot osteoarthropathy in diabetes: a brief review with an emphasis on clinical practice. World J Diabetes 2011;2(5):59–65.
80. Rajbhandari SM, Jenkins RC, Davies C, et al. Charcot neuroarthropathy in diabetes mellitus. Diabetologia 2002;45(8):1085–96.
81. Tesfaye S, Boulton AJ, Dyck PJ, et al. Diabetic neuropathies: update on definitions, diagnostic criteria, estimation of severity, and treatments. Diabetes Care 2010;33(10):2285–93.
82. Schade VL, Andersen CA. A literature-based guide to the conservative and surgical management of the acute Charcot foot and ankle. Diabet Foot Ankle 2015; 6:26627.
83. Schlossbauer T, Mioc T, Sommerey S, et al. Magnetic resonance imaging in early stage charcot arthropathy: correlation of imaging findings and clinical symptoms. Eur J Med Res 2008;13(9):409–14.
84. Chantelau E. The perils of procrastination: effects of early vs. delayed detection and treatment of incipient Charcot fracture. Diabet Med 2005;22(12):1707–12.
85. Chantelau E, Poll LW. Evaluation of the diabetic charcot foot by MR imaging or plain radiography–an observational study. Exp Clin Endocrinol Diabetes 2006; 114(8):428–31.
86. Chantelau E, Richter A, Schmidt-Grigoriadis P, et al. The diabetic charcot foot: MRI discloses bone stress injury as trigger mechanism of neuroarthropathy. Exp Clin Endocrinol Diabetes 2006;114(3):118–23.
87. Pakarinen TK, Laine HJ, Honkonen SE, et al. Charcot arthropathy of the diabetic foot. Current concepts and review of 36 cases. Scand J Surg 2002;91(2): 195–201.
88. Schoots IG, Slim FJ, Busch-Westbroek TE, et al. Neuro-osteoarthropathy of the foot-radiologist: friend or foe? Semin Musculoskelet Radiol 2010;14(3):365–76.
89. Yu GV, Hudson JR. Evaluation and treatment of stage 0 Charcot's neuroarthropathy of the foot and ankle. J Am Podiatr Med Assoc 2002;92(4):210–20.
90. Zampa V, Bargellini I, Rizzo L, et al. Role of dynamic MRI in the follow-up of acute Charcot foot in patients with diabetes mellitus. Skeletal Radiol 2011; 40(8):991–9.
91. Armstrong DG, Peters EJ. Charcot's arthropathy of the foot. J Am Podiatr Med Assoc 2002;92(7):390–4.
92. Perrin BM, Gardner MJ, Suhaimi A, et al. Charcot osteoarthropathy of the foot. Aust Fam Physician 2010;39(3):117–9.

93. Salo PT, Theriault E, Wiley RG. Selective ablation of rat knee joint innervation with injected immunotoxin: a potential new model for the study of neuropathic arthritis. J Orthop Res 1997;15(4):622–8.
94. Tan AL, Greenstein A, Jarrett SJ, et al. Acute neuropathic joint disease: a medical emergency? Diabetes Care 2005;28(12):2962–4.
95. Caputo GM, Ulbrecht J, Cavanagh PR, et al. The Charcot foot in diabetes: six key points. Am Fam Physician 1998;57(11):2705–10.
96. Giurini JM, Chrzan JS, Gibbons GW, et al. Charcot's disease in diabetic patients. Correct diagnosis can prevent progressive deformity. Postgrad Med 1991;89(4):163–9.
97. Shibata T, Tada K, Hashizume C. The results of arthrodesis of the ankle for leprotic neuroarthropathy. J Bone Joint Surg Am 1990;72(5):749–56.
98. Sinacore DR, Withrington NC. Recognition and management of acute neuropathic (Charcot) arthropathies of the foot and ankle. J Orthop Sports Phys Ther 1999;29(12):736–46.
99. Rogers LC, Frykberg RG, Armstrong DG, et al. The Charcot foot in diabetes. J Am Podiatr Med Assoc 2011;101(5):437–46.
100. Pinzur MS, Lio T, Posner M. Treatment of Eichenholtz stage I Charcot foot arthropathy with a weightbearing total contact cast. Foot Ankle Int 2006;27(5): 324–9.
101. Pinzur MS, Shields N, Trepman E, et al. Current practice patterns in the treatment of Charcot foot. Foot Ankle Int 2000;21(11):916–20.
102. Armstrong DG, Todd WF, Lavery LA, et al. The natural history of acute Charcot's arthropathy in a diabetic foot specialty clinic. J Am Podiatr Med Assoc 1997; 87(6):272–8.
103. Pinzur M. Surgical versus accommodative treatment for Charcot arthropathy of the midfoot. Foot Ankle Int 2004;25(8):545–9.
104. Sommer TC, Lee TH. Charcot foot: the diagnostic dilemma. Am Fam Physician 2001;64(9):1591–8.
105. Hastings MK, Sinacore DR, Fielder FA, et al. Bone mineral density during total contact cast immobilization for a patient with neuropathic (Charcot) arthropathy. Phys Ther 2005;85(3):249–56.
106. Richard JL, Almasri M, Schuldiner S. Treatment of acute Charcot foot with bisphosphonates: a systematic review of the literature. Diabetologia 2012;55(5): 1258–64.
107. Lee L, Blume PA, Sumpio B. Charcot joint disease in diabetes mellitus. Ann Vasc Surg 2003;17(5):571–80.
108. Simon SR, Tejwani SG, Wilson DL, et al. Arthrodesis as an early alternative to nonoperative management of charcot arthropathy of the diabetic foot. J Bone Joint Surg Am 2000;82-A(7):939–50.
109. Sella EJ, Barrette C. Staging of Charcot neuroarthropathy along the medial column of the foot in the diabetic patient. J Foot Ankle Surg 1999;38(1):34–40.
110. Stapleton JJ, Zgonis T. Surgical reconstruction of the diabetic Charcot foot: internal, external or combined fixation? Clin Podiatr Med Surg 2012;29(3):425–33.
111. Zgonis T, Roukis TS, Lamm BM. Charcot foot and ankle reconstruction: current thinking and surgical approaches. Clin Podiatr Med Surg 2007;24(3):505–17, ix.
112. Zgonis T, Stapleton JJ, Jeffries LC, et al. Surgical treatment of charcot neuropathy. AORN J 2008;87(5):971–86 [quiz: 987–90].
113. Sammarco VJ. Superconstructs in the treatment of charcot foot deformity: plantar plating, locked plating, and axial screw fixation. Foot Ankle Clin 2009; 14(3):393–407.

114. Sammarco VJ, Sammarco GJ, Walker EW Jr, et al. Midtarsal arthrodesis in the treatment of Charcot midfoot arthropathy. J Bone Joint Surg Am 2009;91(1): 80–91.

115. Grant WP, Garcia-Lavin SE, Sabo RT, et al. A retrospective analysis of 50 consecutive Charcot diabetic salvage reconstructions. J Foot Ankle Surg 2009;48(1):30–8.

116. Pappalardo J, Fitzgerald R. Utilization of advanced modalities in the management of diabetic Charcot neuroarthropathy. J Diabetes Sci Technol 2010;4(5): 1114–20.

117. Camathias C, Valderrabano V, Oberli H. Routine pin tract care in external fixation is unnecessary: a randomised, prospective, blinded controlled study. Injury 2012;43(11):1969–73.

118. Wiewiorski M, Valderrabano V. Intramedullary fixation of the medial column of the foot with a solid bolt in Charcot midfoot arthropathy: a case report. J Foot Ankle Surg 2012;51(3):379–81.

119. Wiewiorski M, Yasui T, Miska M, et al. Solid bolt fixation of the medial column in Charcot midfoot arthropathy. J Foot Ankle Surg 2013;52(1):88–94.

120. Belczyk R, Ramanujam CL, Capobianco CM, et al. Combined midfoot arthrodesis, muscle flap coverage, and circular external fixation for the chronic ulcerated Charcot deformity. Foot Ankle Spec 2010;3(1):40–4.

121. Capobianco CM, Ramanujam CL, Zgonis T. Charcot foot reconstruction with combined internal and external fixation: case report. J Orthop Surg Res 2010; 5:7.

122. Wukich DK, Belczyk RJ, Burns PR, et al. Complications encountered with circular ring fixation in persons with diabetes mellitus. Foot Ankle Int 2008;29(10): 994–1000.

123. Baumhauer J, Pinzur MS, Donahue R, et al. Site selection and pain outcome after autologous bone graft harvest. Foot Ankle Int 2014;35(2):104–7.

124. Deresh GM, Cohen M. Reconstruction of the diabetic Charcot foot incorporating bone grafts. J Foot Ankle Surg 1996;35(5):474–88.

125. Fitzgibbons TC, Hawks MA, McMullen ST, et al. Bone grafting in surgery about the foot and ankle: indications and techniques. J Am Acad Orthop Surg 2011; 19(2):112–20.

126. Roukis T. A simple technique for harvesting autogenous bone grafts from the calcaneus. Foot Ankle Int 2006;27(11):998–9.

127. Roukis TS, Hyer CF, Philbin TM, et al. Complications associated with autogenous bone marrow aspirate harvest from the lower extremity: an observational cohort study. J Foot Ankle Surg 2009;48(6):668–71.

128. Roukis TS, Zgonis T, Tiernan B. Autologous platelet-rich plasma for wound and osseous healing: a review of the literature and commercially available products. Adv Ther 2006;23(2):218–37.

129. Pinzur MS. Use of platelet-rich concentrate and bone marrow aspirate in high-risk patients with Charcot arthropathy of the foot. Foot Ankle Int 2009;30(2): 124–7.

130. Bem R, Jirkovska A, Fejfarova V, et al. Intranasal calcitonin in the treatment of acute Charcot neuroosteoarthropathy: a randomized controlled trial. Diabetes Care 2006;29(6):1392–4.

131. Fourman MS, Borst EW, Bogner E, et al. Recombinant human BMP-2 increases the incidence and rate of healing in complex ankle arthrodesis. Clin Orthop Relat Res 2014;472(2):732–9.

132. Liporace FA, Bibbo C, Azad V, et al. Bioadjuvants for complex ankle and hind-foot reconstruction. Foot Ankle Clin 2007;12(1):75–106.

133. Anderson CL, Whitaker MC. Heterotopic ossification associated with recombinant human bone morphogenetic protein-2 (infuse) in posterolateral lumbar spine fusion: a case report. Spine (Phila Pa 1976) 2012;37(8):E502–6.

134. Burkus JK, Dryer RF, Peloza JH. Retrograde ejaculation following single-level anterior lumbar surgery with or without recombinant human bone morphogenetic protein-2 in 5 randomized controlled trials: clinical article. J Neurosurg Spine 2013;18(2):112–21.

135. Slater GL, Sayres SC, O'Malley MJ. Anterior ankle arthrodesis. World J Orthop 2014;5(1):1–5.

136. Loiselle AE, Kelly M, Hammert WC. Biological augmentation of flexor tendon repair: a challenging cellular landscape. J Hand Surg 2016;41(1):144–9 [quiz: 149].

137. Soldatis JJ, Goodfellow DB, Wilber JH. End-to-end operative repair of Achilles tendon rupture. Am J Sports Med 1997;25(1):90–5.

138. Kannus P, Jozsa L. Histopathological changes preceding spontaneous rupture of a tendon. A controlled study of 891 patients. J Bone Joint Surg Am 1991; 73(10):1507–25.

139. Bestwick CS, Maffulli N. Reactive oxygen species and tendinopathy: do they matter? Br J Sports Med 2004;38(6):672–4.

140. Zhang J, Wang JH. Production of PGE(2) increases in tendons subjected to repetitive mechanical loading and induces differentiation of tendon stem cells into non-tenocytes. J Orthop Res 2010;28(2):198–203.

141. Li Z, Yang G, Khan M, et al. Inflammatory response of human tendon fibroblasts to cyclic mechanical stretching. Am J Sports Med 2004;32(2):435–40.

142. Flick J, Devkota A, Tsuzaki M, et al. Cyclic loading alters biomechanical properties and secretion of PGE2 and NO from tendon explants. Clin Biomech (Bristol, Avon) 2006;21(1):99–106.

143. Tsuzaki M, Guyton G, Garrett W, et al. IL-1 beta induces COX2, MMP-1, -3 and -13, ADAMTS-4, IL-1 beta and IL-6 in human tendon cells. J Orthop Res 2003;21(2): 256–64.

144. Bidell MR, Lodise TP. Fluoroquinolone-Associated Tendinopathy: Does Levofloxacin Pose the Greatest Risk? Pharmacotherapy 2016;36(6):679–93.

145. Arabyat RM, Raisch DW, McKoy JM, et al. Fluoroquinolone-associated tendon-rupture: a summary of reports in the Food and Drug Administration's adverse event reporting system. Expert Opin Drug Saf 2015;14(11):1653–60.

146. Corps AN, Harrall RL, Curry VA, et al. Ciprofloxacin enhances the stimulation of matrix metalloproteinase 3 expression by interleukin-1beta in human tendon-derived cells. A potential mechanism of fluoroquinolone-induced tendinopathy. Arthritis Rheum 2002;46(11):3034–40.

147. Mobasheri A, Shakibaei M. Is tendinitis an inflammatory disease initiated and driven by pro-inflammatory cytokines such as interleukin 1beta? Histol Histopathol 2013;28(8):955–64.

148. Andersson C, Odensten M, Good L, et al. Surgical or non-surgical treatment of acute rupture of the anterior cruciate ligament. A randomized study with long-term follow-up. J Bone Joint Surg Am 1989;71(7):965–74.

149. Nagineni CN, Amiel D, Green MH, et al. Characterization of the intrinsic properties of the anterior cruciate and medial collateral ligament cells: an in vitro cell culture study. J Orthop Res 1992;10(4):465–75.

150. Woo SL, Vogrin TM, Abramowitch SD. Healing and repair of ligament injuries in the knee. J Am Acad Orthop Surg 2000;8(6):364–72.

151. Juneja SC, Schwarz EM, O'Keefe RJ, et al. Cellular and molecular factors in flexor tendon repair and adhesions: a histological and gene expression analysis. Connect Tissue Res 2013;54(3):218–26.

152. Manning CN, Havlioglu N, Knutsen E, et al. The early inflammatory response after flexor tendon healing: a gene expression and histological analysis. J Orthop Res 2014;32(5):645–52.

153. Brophy RH, Tycksen ED, Sandell LJ, et al. Changes in transcriptome-wide gene expression of anterior cruciate ligament tears based on time from injury. Am J Sports Med 2016;44(8):2064–75.

154. Chaudhury S, Xia Z, Thakkar D, et al. Gene expression profiles of changes underlying different-sized human rotator cuff tendon tears. J Shoulder Elbow Surg 2016. [Epub ahead of print].

155. Lilly SI, Messer TM. Complications after treatment of flexor tendon injuries. J Am Acad Orthop Surg 2006;14(7):387–96.

156. Dy CJ, Hernandez-Soria A, Ma Y, et al. Complications after flexor tendon repair: a systematic review and meta-analysis. J Hand Surg 2012;37(3):543–51.e541.

157. Hasslund S, Jacobson JA, Dadali T, et al. Adhesions in a murine flexor tendon graft model: autograft versus allograft reconstruction. J Orthop Res 2008;26(6): 824–33.

158. Tan V, Nourbakhsh A, Capo J, et al. Effects of nonsteroidal anti-inflammatory drugs on flexor tendon adhesion. J Hand Surg 2010;35(6):941–7.

159. Thomopoulos S, Genin GM, Galatz LM. The development and morphogenesis of the tendon-to-bone insertion - what development can teach us about healing. J Musculoskelet Neuronal Interact 2010;10(1):35–45.

160. Benjamin M, Evans EJ, Copp L. The histology of tendon attachments to bone in man. J Anat 1986;149:89–100.

161. Doschak MR, Zernicke RF. Structure, function and adaptation of bone-tendon and bone-ligament complexes. J Musculoskelet Neuronal Interact 2005;5(1): 35–40.

162. Benjamin M, McGonagle D. Entheses: tendon and ligament attachment sites. Scand J Med Sci Sports 2009;19(4):520–7.

163. Trotter JA. Structure-function considerations of muscle-tendon junctions. Comp Biochem Physiol A Mol Integr Physiol 2002;133(4):1127–33.

164. Ahmad J, Repka M, Raikin SM. Treatment of myotendinous Achilles ruptures. Foot Ankle Int 2013;34(8):1074–8.

165. Liu SH, Panossian V, al-Shaikh R, et al. Morphology and matrix composition during early tendon to bone healing. Clin Orthop Relat Res 1997;(339):253–60.

166. Thomopoulos S, Williams GR, Soslowsky LJ. Tendon to bone healing: differences in biomechanical, structural, and compositional properties due to a range of activity levels. J Biomech Eng 2003;125(1):106–13.

167. de la Durantaye M, Piette AB, van Rooijen N, et al. Macrophage depletion reduces cell proliferation and extracellular matrix accumulation but increases the ultimate tensile strength of injured Achilles tendons. J Orthop Res 2014; 32(2):279–85.

168. Freedman BR, Sarver JJ, Buckley MR, et al. Biomechanical and structural response of healing Achilles tendon to fatigue loading following acute injury. J Biomech 2014;47(9):2028–34.

169. Godbout C, Bilodeau R, Van Rooijen N, et al. Transient neutropenia increases macrophage accumulation and cell proliferation but does not improve repair following intratendinous rupture of Achilles tendon. J Orthop Res 2010;28(8): 1084–91.

170. Xia W, Wang Y, Appleyard RC, et al. Spontaneous recovery of injured Achilles tendon in inducible nitric oxide synthase gene knockout mice. Inflamm Res 2006;55(1):40–5.
171. Chhabra A, Tsou D, Clark RT, et al. GDF-5 deficiency in mice delays Achilles tendon healing. J Orthop Res 2003;21(5):826–35.
172. Palmes D, Spiegel HU, Schneider TO, et al. Achilles tendon healing: long-term biomechanical effects of postoperative mobilization and immobilization in a new mouse model. J Orthop Res 2002;20(5):939–46.
173. Juneja SC, Veillette C. Defects in tendon, ligament, and enthesis in response to genetic alterations in key proteoglycans and glycoproteins: a review. Arthritis 2013;2013:154812.
174. Branford OA, Klass BR, Grobbelaar AO, et al. The growth factors involved in flexor tendon repair and adhesion formation. J Hand Surg Eur 2014;39(1): 60–70.
175. Rawson S, Cartmell S, Wong J. Suture techniques for tendon repair; a comparative review. Muscles Ligaments Tendons J 2013;3(3):220–8.
176. Dimmen S. Effects of Cox inhibitors on bone and tendon healing. Acta Orthop Suppl 2011;82(342):1–22.
177. Dimmen S, Nordsletten L, Engebretsen L, et al. The effect of parecoxib and indometacin on tendon-to-bone healing in a bone tunnel: an experimental study in rats. J Bone Joint Surg Br 2009;91(2):259–63.
178. Carlstedt CA, Madsen K, Wredmark T. The influence of indomethacin on tendon healing. A biomechanical and biochemical study. Arch Orthop Trauma Surg 1986;105(6):332–6.
179. Forslund C, Bylander B, Aspenberg P. Indomethacin and celecoxib improve tendon healing in rats. Acta Orthop Scand 2003;74(4):465–9.
180. Dakin SG, Dudhia J, Smith RK. Resolving an inflammatory concept: the importance of inflammation and resolution in tendinopathy. Vet Immunol Immunopathol 2014;158(3–4):121–7.
181. Bissell L, Tibrewal S, Sahni V, et al. Growth factors and platelet rich plasma in anterior cruciate ligament reconstruction. Curr Stem Cel Res Ther 2014;10(1): 19–25.
182. Farhat YM, Al-Maliki AA, Easa A, et al. TGF-beta1 suppresses plasmin and MMP activity in flexor tendon cells via PAI-1: implications for scarless flexor tendon repair. J Cell Physiol 2015;230(2):318–26.
183. Davis ME, Gumucio JP, Sugg KB, et al. MMP inhibition as a potential method to augment the healing of skeletal muscle and tendon extracellular matrix. J Appl Physiol (1985) 2013;115(6):884–91.
184. Wong R, Alam N, McGrouther AD, et al. Tendon grafts: their natural history, biology and future development. J Hand Surg Eur 2015;40(7):669–81.
185. Galatz LM, Gerstenfeld L, Heber-Katz E, et al. Tendon regeneration and scar formation: the concept of scarless healing. J Orthop Res 2015;33(6):823–31.

The Efficacy of Platelet-Derived Growth Factor as a Bone-Stimulating Agent

 CrossMark

Ethan S. Krell, MBS[a,1], Christopher W. DiGiovanni, MD[b,*]

KEYWORDS

- Bone graft substitute • Foot and ankle arthrodesis • Fusion
- Platelet-derived growth factor • rhPDGF-BB

KEY POINTS

- The use of recombinant human platelet-derived growth factor (PDGF)-BB/β-tricalcium phosphate has been approved in 2015 by the Food and Drug Administration (FDA) as an alternative to autograft during ankle and hindfoot fusion surgery.
- Augment Bone Graft upregulates osteoblast and blood vessel formation, which promotes chondrogenesis/osteogenesis at the fusion area of interest.
- In a phase III randomized, controlled trial, 66.5% of PDGF-treated joints and 62.6% of autograft-treated joints demonstrated fusion on computed tomography scanning at 24 weeks postoperatively.
- Clinical success was deemed directly dependent on good surgical technique, ensuring that bony contact between any joint surfaces intended for fusion was maximized while not impairing direct host bone apposition.

INTRODUCTION

Since the latter one-half of the 20th century, foot and ankle surgeons have focused on achieving rigid fixation to achieve successful arthrodesis. Alarmingly, however, more recent investigations have identified numerous risk factors capable of impairing osseous healing (diabetes, osteoporosis, tobacco use, age, corticosteroid therapy, and various pharmaceutical agents) and threatening the capacity to achieve uneventful fusion across diseased articular surfaces—even in the presence of a stable

---

Disclosure Statement: C.W. DiGiovanni is a paid consultant for Wright Medical Technologies, and has also received research funding for comparative study of Augment Bone Graft versus Autogenous Bone Graft. E.S. Krell has nothing to disclose.
[a] Department of Orthopaedics, Rutgers New Jersey Medical School, Newark, NJ, USA;
[b] Division of Foot and Ankle Surgery, Department of Orthopaedic Surgery, Massachusetts General Hospital, Harvard Medical School, 55 Fruit Street, Boston, MA 02114, USA
[1] Present address: 10 Barchester Way, Westfield, NJ 07090.
* Corresponding author.
E-mail address: CWDiGiovanni@MGH.Harvard.edu

mechanical environment. Reported delayed and nonunion rates within these high-risk populations have averaged approximately 10%, but ranged as high as 40%.[1–3] In response to these findings, the past decade has ushered in a new era of orthobiologic research aimed at optimizing the healing environment during fusion surgery: focus has shifted from looking not just at the mechanical but also at the biological nature of these procedures. Specifically, recent advances in cellular and protein technology have led to the development of cutting edge growth factors and related biologic agents, which can serve as useful adjuncts to conventional therapies by promoting an elevated level of bone and soft tissue healing in this higher risk patient population. Platelet-derived growth factor (PDGF) represents a particular bone-stimulating agent of recent clinical interest that has proven effective for foot and ankle surgical patients through well-controlled, level I clinical evidence. It is likely that this protein technology will have a major positive impact on the future care of patients requiring hindfoot or ankle fusion procedures.

PDGF refers to a family of proteins that are released from platelets and macrophages in response to tissue injury and bone fracture.[4,5] The PDGF-BB dimer has been found to be the most potent form of the growth factor, and is both chemotactic and mitogenic for osteoblast progenitor cells as well as osteoblasts (the key bone-forming cell).[6,7] In addition, PDGF-BB has the capacity to promote new blood vessel formation (angiogenesis) even in the proximity of compromised host tissues, which allows for an influx of proinflammatory and chondrogenic/osteogenic agents to the fusion area of interest.[8] Based on more than a decade of rigorous basic science, animal, and human clinical research, the use of recombinant human PDGF-BB (rhPDGF-BB) in conjunction with a β-tricalcium phosphate (β-TCP) carrier (Augment Bone Graft, Wright Medical Technology, Inc., Memphis, TN) was approved in 2015 by the Food and Drug Administration (FDA) as a viable alternative to autograft in ankle and hindfoot fusion surgery. This therapy has already been available for commercial use and used quite successfully in Canada since 2009, Australia (2011), and New Zealand (2011). Alternative applications of rhPDGF-BB for bone defects in dental patients as well as for wound healing in neuropathic ulceration are also FDA approved. We aim to review the key preclinical and clinical trials leading to the approval of rhPDGF-BB for use in the foot and ankle surgical population.

PRECLINICAL INVESTIGATION

Between 1989 and 2009, several animal studies demonstrated the usefulness of rhPDGF-BB in potentiating bone healing. Al-Zube and colleagues,[9] examined the effect of intramedullary rhPDGF-BB treatment on femoral fracture healing in diabetic rats. An increase in early cellular proliferation was noted within the fracture callus of experimental rats as compared with controls. Further, rhPDGF-BB treatment increased the maximum torque to failure at 8 weeks after fracture and resulted in a greater callus bone area at 12 weeks after fracture. Similarly, Hollinger and colleagues[10] found a significant increase in torsional strength of fractured tibiae 5 weeks after rhPDGF-BB administration in geriatric, osteoporotic rats. The healed fractures and contralateral (nonfractured) tibiae had equivalent biomechanical properties at the 5-week time point. Additionally, local rhPDGF-BB treatment accelerated bone growth in a rabbit osteotomy model,[11] increased lumbar bone mineral density in baboons,[12] and enhanced bone healing in a rat model of distraction osteogenesis.[13] Local rhPDGF-BB, in combination with insulinlike growth factor-1, has also been shown to increase osseointegration of dental implants in a beagle dog model as well as promote bone regeneration of periodontal osseous defects in humans.[14–16]

ANKLE AND HINDFOOT ARTHRODESIS

Ankle or hindfoot arthrodesis is indicated for the treatment of recalcitrant arthritis, deformity, or instability affecting these joints as a result of trauma, infection, primary osteoarthritis, rheumatologic or crystalline conditions, and other associated maladies that can affect this anatomy—especially in adults 50 years or older.[17] In 2014, more than 80,000 fusions were performed and there were 50,000 new cases of end-stage arthritis. Nonunion has, over the past century, been one of the most feared complications after ankle or hindfoot arthrodesis. Despite lack of sufficient evidence to support anything beyond a grade C recommendation in recent years, autologous bone graft (ABG) has long been heralded as the gold standard for combating nonunion.[18] Although still considered over the past century as our most effective healing adjunct, it has not been without its shortcomings. ABG remains limited in quantity and can be associated with significant harvest site pain as well as additional surgical morbidity.[18,19] Further, the quality of ABG varies significantly based on site of harvest, even within the same patient.[20,21] Use of alternative bone-stimulating agents obtained through recombinant technology such as rhPDGF-BB/β-TCP (Augment Bone Graft) offers the potential to avoid any need for additional surgery to harvest autograft. Agents such as rhPDGF-BB/β-TCP have also documented a well-described safety profile and a much more predictable pharmacokinetics (dose–response efficacy). In the future, these differences may serve to offer major advantages to foot and ankle patients during elective fusion surgery. Herein we review the clinical evidence regarding the use of Augment Bone Graft in the ankle and hindfoot.

Daniels and colleagues[22] conducted a prospective trial in Canada with a single cohort group to evaluate the efficacy of rhPDGF-BB in 60 patients undergoing ankle, hindfoot, or midfoot arthrodesis. rhPDGF-BB is composed of 0.3 mg/mL of rhPDGF-BB combined with β-TCP (a scaffold that acts as a framework for bone growth). Use of computed tomography (CT) scanning revealed at least 50% bridging across the fusion site(s) in 43% of patients after 6 weeks, and 75% after 12 to 16 weeks. Radiographic union was apparent in 52 of 59 patients (88%) by 36 weeks postoperatively. These results are comparable with ankle and hindfoot fusion rates in patients receiving ABG.[1,17]

A US pilot study[23] in 2011 became the first randomized, controlled trial evaluating PDGF in foot and ankle surgery. Patients undergoing ankle and hindfoot arthrodesis were randomized prospectively to receive either rhPDGF-BB/β-TCP (n = 13) or ABG (n = 6). After 12 weeks, radiographic union was achieved in 43% of patients in the PDGF group compared with 33% in the ABG group. A 12-week CT scan showed 50% or greater healing in 9 of 13 PDGF patients (69%) and 3 of 6 ABG patients (50%). Radiographic union at 36 weeks after surgery was apparent in 10 of 13 cases (77%) and 3 of 6 cases (50%) for PDGF versus ABG, respectively. No serious adverse events were reported in either patient group of the study, although patients in the ABG group were found to have increased operative/anesthetic times.

In the subsequent phase III FDA randomized, controlled clinical trial,[24] 434 patients requiring ankle or hindfoot arthrodesis were enrolled 2:1 to prospectively receive either rhPDGF-BB/β- TCP (260 patients; 394 joints) or ABG (137 patients; 203 joints). The primary endpoint was 24-week CT scanning across all fusion sites, with successful fusion defined as requiring more than 50% osseous bridging—as determined by an independent, blinded radiologist. Two types of CT scan assessments were performed to account for patients with multiple fusion sites. The full complement analysis defined successful arthrodesis as fusion at all joints, whereas the all joints analysis assessed each joint independently. After 6 months, the full complement analysis fusion rate was

61.2% for patients in the PDGF group, compared with 62.0% for those in the ABG group ($P = .038$; statistically noninferior). A total of 66.5% PDGF-treated joints and 62.6% ABG-treated joints demonstrated fusion on CT scan ($P<.001$; noninferiority). At the 6-month time point, nonunion or delayed union was observed in 9.2% of joints in PDGF group versus 10.9% in the ABG group ($P<.001$; noninferiority). Notably, harvest site pain and morbidity was reported only by patients having been treated with ABG. Moreover, at 6 months, 0% of PDGF-treated patients and 12.7% of ABG-treated patients reported chronic pain at the autograft donor site ($P<.001$; superiority), with 9.2% still experiencing pain after a full year of follow-up ($P<.001$; superiority). Multiple clinical and functional outcomes were found to be statistically equivalent between the 2 groups, including the Foot Function Index total score, American Orthopaedic Foot and Ankle Society total score, and ShortForm-12 Physical Component Score.

CT scans confirmed that better fusion outcomes ($\geq$50% graft material at 9 weeks) resulted in better improvement in patient outcomes ($\geq$50% osseous bridging at 24 weeks) and that fusion success was directly related to graft fill. Of the reviewed joints, 82% had a 50% or greater graft fill in the fusion space, whereas 18% of reviewed joints had less than 50% graft fill in the fusion space. Of the joints with 50% or greater graft fill, 81.1% showed fusion success at week 24. In contrast, in joints with less than 50% graft fill, the rate of fusion success was only 20.8%. Further, 89.8% of joints with 50% or greater graft fill showed clinical healing at week 24 in contrast with 72.3% clinical healing at week 24 in joints with less than 50% graft fill.

SURGICAL TECHNIQUE

The ideal surgical technique using Augment Bone Graft has been optimized over the course of a 7-year experience with sequential clinical trials and incorporation of extensive feedback from experienced, fellowship-trained foot and ankle surgeons across North America. All of the human trials referenced included these individuals, and protocols were standardized across each investigation. Based on this extensive research, there are several key principles to keep in mind when using Augment Bone Graft for foot and ankle fusion surgery. The most important finding to garner from these data is that optimized use of this (as well as any) graft material means maximizing bony contact area—but not doing so at the expense of direct host bone apposition. This means that the surgeon should avoid any unopposed surface irregularity across the entire joint surface area to be fused to maximize available contact area for healing; thus, all voids, small cysts, and any other defects should be packed with graft material to a level that corresponds with the surface of any adjacently prepared normal host bone—but not beyond this point. The point to be emphasized is that overstuffing the joint with graft in any manner that impairs direct contact of all unaffected innate host bone surfaces is counterproductive, and should be avoided. These points will be elaborated further, including an adaptation of the surgical techniques originally described for all investigators to follow in the clinical trials.

As with all fusion operations of the foot and ankle, initial exposure is predicated on the areas of interest to be fused using standard, well-described approaches. After identification of the intended fusion site, the surgeon should debride and denude any remaining articular cartilage or scar to promote maximal exposure of all viable host bone on both sides of each joint being prepared for arthrodesis (**Fig. 1**). It is recommended that these surfaces thereafter also be decorticated with the use of an osteotome, burr, drill, curette, and/or rongeur to maximize an osseous healing response and allow ultimate apposition of healthy, vascularized bone (**Fig. 2**A). Optimization of blood flow to the fusion site can be improved by either feathering and/or

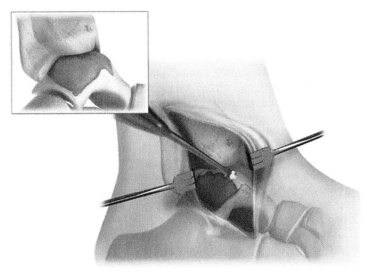

Fig. 1. Debridement. After fully exposing the joint to be fused all remaining cartilage is removed and the bone is denuded of tissue to reveal the osseous surfaces. (*From* Surgical Technique Augment Bone Graft. Memphis [TN]: Wright Medical Technology, Inc.; 2015.)

perforating the subchondral plate of each articular surface intended for arthrodesis using any combination of the aforementioned instruments (**Fig. 2**B). All of this preparation should be done before placement of the Augment Bone Graft material. Once formal joint preparation has been completed, the surgeon should thoroughly irrigate and then remove any debris or residual fluid that might remain in the area of fusion. Before Augment Bone Graft implantation, it is then recommended that the surgeon appose each of the articular host surfaces intended for fusion to inspect for any areas of poor or incomplete contact. Cortical and articular irregularities are almost always present in these patients, and it is important to identify these locations because they will represent the primary sites of Augment Bone Graft incorporation. Immediately after this inspection, the surgeon should request the expected volume of Augment Bone Graft be sterilely opened and mixed on the back table. This mixture of rhPDGF and β-TCP must saturate for at least 10 minutes before implantation for maximal

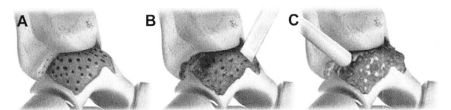

Fig. 2. Subchondral exposure and application of graft. The cortical bone may be perforated with a drill (*A*) or subchondral exposure can be achieved with a burr, osteotome or curette to "feather" the joint surface (*B*). Either technique can be performed to maximize the surface area of bleeding bone before application of the graft (*C*). The bone graft is placed wherever there is not direct host bone to host bone apposition. (*Adapted from* Surgical Technique Augment Bone Graft. Memphis [TN]: Wright Medical Technology, Inc.; 2015.)

effect. The product consists of 2 primary components: β-TCP granules approximating 1000 to 2000 μm and rhPDGF-BB solution at a concentration of 0.3 mg/mL.

Once the location and depth of all surface irregularities has been determined, the surgeon must then take the rhPDGF-BB immersed β-TCP and, with the use of a small curette or scoop, pack the Augment Bone Graft directly into, not around, all these particular bony defects throughout both sides of the joint intended for arthrodesis (**Fig. 2**C). Once this has been completed, the surgeon can then re-oppose the surfaces to ensure placement of Augment Bone Graft wherever there is still gapping (indirect host bone to host bone apposition). Care should also be taken to ensure that all Augment Bone Graft material is contained within the confines of these defects; graft should not be permitted to extend beyond the perimeter of the joint surface or beyond the surrounding soft tissue capsule. It should be noted that Augment Bone Graft is designed only for use in open orthopedic surgical procedures of the foot or ankle. Efficacy in other parts of the musculoskeletal system or as an adjunct to arthroscopic procedures has yet to be studied sufficiently.

Once apposition has been optimized at all sites of intended fusion, the surgeon should proceed with routine rigid, anatomic reduction and fixation using implants based on individual preference. After this step, each fusion site should then be immersed at its periphery with any remaining rhPDGF-BB liquid solution (**Fig. 3**). Care should be taken not to irrigate any of these areas until each joint capsule is closed completely, to avoid unintentional dilution of the Augment Bone Graft. It is further recommended that this portion of the procedure be performed under tourniquet control, so that dilution by irrigation or bleeding can be avoided until meticulous periosteal closure has occurred. After a carefully layered capsular and soft tissue closure of each joint space to contain all graft material at its intended site, routine splinting and any remaining surgical or postoperative protocols can be performed.

SUMMARY

As recombinant technology continues to advance, a growing body of literature suggests that perhaps ABG is no longer the optimal grafting material for complex

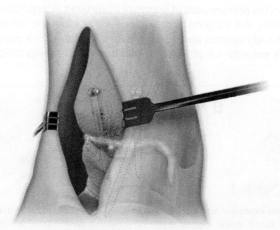

Fig. 3. Application of the remaining graft. After reduction and rigid fixation is achieved, any remaining graft is packed around the fused joint and careful closure is performed to ensure the graft is contained within the joint space. (*From* Surgical Technique Augment Bone Graft. Memphis [TN]: Wright Medical Technology, Inc.; 2015.)

orthopedic surgical procedures. Augment Bone Graft represents a level I evidence-based alternative capable of facilitating fusion success equivalent to ABG during ankle or hindfoot arthrodesis, while avoiding the subsequent donor site pain and other potential complications associated with autologous graft harvest. Since 2009, this promising growth factor therapy has been used extensively outside of the United States, with great success. As these data suggest, proper surgical technique is essential to maximize Augment Bone Graft's healing capacity. Orthobiologic therapy aims to enhance the body's natural healing response after damage to bone, tendons, cartilage, and ligaments and in conditions that impair musculoskeletal regeneration. Continued research will likely uncover additional alternatives to improve our current armamentarium of orthopedic therapies.

REFERENCES

1. Easley ME, Trnka HJ, Schon LC, et al. Isolated subtalar arthrodesis. J Bone Joint Surg Am 2000;82:613–24.
2. Frey C, Halikus NM, Vu-Rose T, et al. A review of ankle arthrodesis: predisposing factors to nonunion. Foot Ankle Int 1994;15:581–4.
3. Kagel EM, Einhorn TA. Alterations of fracture healing in the diabetic condition. Iowa Orthop J 1996;16:147–52.
4. Andrew JG, Hoyland JA, Freemont AJ, et al. Platelet-derived growth factor expression in normally healing human fractures. Bone 1995;16:455–60.
5. Fujii H, Kitazawa R, Maeda S, et al. Expression of platelet-derived growth factor proteins and their receptor alpha and beta mRNAs during fracture healing in the normal mouse. Histochem Cell Biol 1999;112:131–8.
6. Fiedler J, Roderer G, Gunther KP, et al. BMP-2, BMP-4, and PDGF-bb stimulate chemotactic migration of primary human mesenchymal progenitor cells. J Cell Biochem 2002;87:305–12.
7. Tanaka H, Liang CT. Effect of platelet-derived growth factor on DNA synthesis and gene expression in bone marrow stromal cells derived from adult and old rats. J Cell Physiol 1995;164:367–75.
8. Guo P, Hu B, Gu W, et al. Platelet-derived growth factor-B enhances glioma angiogenesis by stimulating vascular endothelial growth factor expression in tumor endothelia and by promoting pericyte recruitment. Am J Pathol 2003;162(4): 1083–93.
9. Al-Zube L, Breitbart EA, O'Connor JP, et al. Recombinant human platelet-derived growth factor BB (rhPDGF-BB) and beta-tricalcium phosphate/collagen matrix enhance fracture healing in a diabetic rat model. J Orthop Res 2009;27(8): 1074–81.
10. Hollinger JO, Onikepe AO, MacKrell J, et al. Accelerated fracture healing in the geriatric, osteoporotic rat with recombinant human platelet-derived growth factor-BB and an injectable beta-tricalcium phosphate/collagen matrix. J Orthop Res 2008;26(1):83–90.
11. Nash TJ, Howlett CR, Martin C, et al. Effect of platelet-derived growth factor on tibial osteotomies in rabbits. Bone 1994;15:203–8.
12. Perrien DS, Young CS, Alvarez-Urena PP, et al. Percutaneous injection of augment injectable bone graft (rhPDGF-BB and beta-tricalcium phosphate [beta-TCP]/bovine type I collagen matrix) increases vertebral bone mineral density in geriatric female baboons. Spine J 2013;13(5):580–6.

13. Moore DC, Ehrlich MG, McAllister SC, et al. Recombinant human platelet-derived growth factor-BB augmentation of new-bone formation in a rat model of distraction osteogenesis. J Bone Joint Surg Am 2009;91(8):1973–84.
14. Lynch SE, Williams RC, Polson AM, et al. A combination of platelet-derived and insulin-like growth factors enhances periodontal regeneration. J Clin Periodontol 1989;16:545–8.
15. Lynch SE, Buser D, Hernandez RA, et al. Effects of the platelet-derived growth factor/insulin-like growth factor-I combination on bone regeneration around titanium dental implants. Results of a pilot study in beagle dogs. J Periodontol 1991;62(11):710–6.
16. Howell TH, Fiorellini JP, Paquette DW, et al. A phase I/II clinical trial to evaluate a combination of recombinant human platelet-derived growth factor-BB and recombinant human insulin-like growth factor-I in patients with periodontal disease. J Periodontol 1997;68(12):1186–93.
17. Haddad SL, Coetzee JC, Estok R, et al. Intermediate and long-term outcomes of total ankle arthroplasty and ankle arthrodesis. A systematic review of the literature. J Bone Joint Surg Am 2007;89(9):1899–905.
18. Lareau CR, Deren ME, Fantry A, et al. Does autogenous bone graft work? A logistic regression analysis of data from 159 papers in the foot and ankle literature. Foot Ankle Surg 2015;21:150–9.
19. DeOrio JK, Farber DC. Morbidity associated with anterior iliac crest bone grafting in foot and ankle surgery. Foot Ankle Int 2005;26:147–51.
20. Chiodo CP, Hahne J, Wilson MG, et al. Histological differences in iliac and tibial bone graft. Foot Ankle Int 2010;31:418–22.
21. Sagi HC, Young ML, Gerstenfeld L, et al. Qualitative and quantitative differences between bone graft obtained from the medullary canal (with a Reamer/Irrigator/Aspirator) and the iliac crest of the same patient. J Bone Joint Surg Am 2012; 94:2128–35.
22. Daniels T, DiGiovanni C, Lau JT, et al. Prospective clinical pilot trial in a single cohort group of rhPDGF in foot arthrodeses. Foot Ankle Int 2010;31:473–9.
23. Digiovanni CW, Baumhauer J, Lin SS, et al. Prospective, randomized, multi-center feasibility trial of rhPDGF-BB versus autologous bone graft in a foot and ankle fusion model. Foot Ankle Int 2011;32(4):344–54.
24. DiGiovanni CW, Lin SS, Baumhauer JF, et al. Recombinant human platelet-derived growth factor-BB and beta-tricalcium phosphate (rhPDGF-BB/beta-TCP): an alternative to autogenous bone graft. J Bone Joint Surg Am 2013; 95(13):1184–92.

Vancouver Experience of Recombinant Human Platelet-Derived Growth Factor

⊕ CrossMark

Alistair Younger, MD[a],*, Murray Penner, MD[b],
Harvey E. Montijo, MD[a]

KEYWORDS

- Foot and ankle arthrodesis • Fusion • PDGF, Platelet-derived growth factor
- Recombinant human platelet-derived growth factor • Bone graft substitute

KEY POINTS

- Joint arthrodesis utilizing autogenous bone graft remains the gold standard of treatment in fusion procedures of the foot and ankle.
- Graft harvest however has been associated with increased morbidity to patients as well as increased costs.
- With this in mind, multiple clinical studies have evaluated the efficacy of recombinant human platelet-derived growth factor (rh-PDGF-BB) with beta-tricalcium phosphate (B-TCP) as an augment in foot and ankle arthrodesis with favorable results.
- These factors have led to the increased use of rh-PDGF-BB with B-TCP here in Vancouver with good clinical results.

BACKGROUND

Arthrodesis is the standard of treatment utilized for end-stage arthritis in foot and ankle surgery. In the United States alone, over 100,000 ankle arthrodesis procedures were performed in 2009.[1] However, nonunions and delayed unions that result in significant morbidity and mortality to patients remain at approximately 10% for ankle arthrodesis based on a recent meta-analysis.[2] These nonunions and delayed unions result in significant morbidity and mortality for patients.[2–4]

The gold standard to assist bone healing in fusion is autogenous bone graft, which has been utilized extensively in arthrodesis procedures.[5,6] The utilization of

Financial Disclosure: Dr A. Younger is a consultant with Wright Medical and previously Biomimetics with no stock options. He has received funding for prior research studies. Dr M. Penner is a consultant for Wright Medical with no stock options. Dr H.E. Montijo has nothing to disclose.
[a] Department of Orthopedics, University of British Columbia, 560-1144 Burrard Street, Vancouver, British Columbia V6Z 2A5, Canada; [b] Department of Orthopedics, University of British Columbia, 1000-1200 Burrard Street, Vancouver, British Columbia V6Z 2C7, Canada
* Corresponding author.
E-mail address: asyounger@shaw.ca

Foot Ankle Clin N Am 21 (2016) 771–776
http://dx.doi.org/10.1016/j.fcl.2016.07.009
1083-7515/16/© 2016 Elsevier Inc. All rights reserved.

foot.theclinics.com

autogenous bone graft is attributed to its osteogenic, osteoinductive, and osteocon-ductive properties.[7] Although considered to be an effective adjuvant treatment to aid in bone healing, complications remain as high as 23% in the recent literature.[8] Com-plications of the harvest site include blood loss, postoperative pain, risk of infection, heterotopic bone formation, nerve injury, hernia, seroma formation, and scarring.[8–10] Although initially felt to be a cost-effective treatment, multiple studies have examined the costs associated with autogenous bone graft harvest. The economic impact ranges anywhere from $2365 to $4154 when one factors in the additional operating room time necessary and additional hospital days utilized.[11–13] Additionally, the quality and quantity of autograft harvested can vary based on patient age, body mass index, sex, overall health status, and the location of harvest.[14]

Current goals consist of finding an adjuvant treatment that provides the benefits of autogenous bone graft without the limitations; recent literature has focused on suitable alternatives. Recombinant human platelet-derived growth factor (rh-PDGF-BB) in combination with an osteoconductive scaffold (beta-tricalcium phos-phate [B-TCP]) is 1 such alternative that promotes bone healing in foot and ankle arthrodesis.[6,15]

CLINICAL BACKGROUND

A prospective, open-label, multicenter study, the Canadian Registration Trial was designed to evaluate rh-PDGF-BB in a calcium phosphate matrix with the primary goal of determining its safety and efficacy. Sixty patients were enrolled in 3 Cana-dian institutions after approval by Health Canada.[16] A cohort study, all patients received rhPDGF-BB with B-TCP and were monitored clinically and radiographi-cally for 9 months. Computed tomography (CT) scans were obtained at 6 and 12 weeks postoperatively, with an optional CT scan at 16 weeks if clinically necessary.

Fifty-nine of 60 patients completed the study. Of these, 37 presented with at least 1 risk factor for nonunion. These included recent smoking history, diabetes, and revi-sion surgery. At 36 weeks, 52 of 59 (88%) patients had radiographic union on plain radiographs. At the 12- to 16-week time period, over 75% of patients exhibited greater than 50% osseous bridging on CT scan. Six (10%) of patients were clinical failures with the recommendation made for revision surgery within 12 months of the index procedure. Moreover, 5 of the 6 patients required revisions of failed mid-foot arthrodesis. Of the 60 patients, zero reported adverse events, and its safety justified pursuit of randomized controlled studies comparing rhPDGF-BB with auto-graft. This study also demonstrated the need to correctly pack the fusion site. Over-stuffing with TCP granules may result in destabilizing the fusion site and might contribute to the nonunion.

With the safety and efficacy of rh-PDGF-BB with B-TCP established, a multicenter, prospective randomized control study directly comparing rh-PDGF with B-TCP to autograft in hindfoot and ankle arthrodesis was performed. Patients were randomized in a 2 to 1 fashion, receiving either rh-PDGF-BB with B-TCP or autograft utilizing rigid fixation. With 434 patients enrolled, fusion was defined as greater than 50% of osseous bridging at 24 weeks. A noninferiority model, results showed the CT fusion rate of autograft and rh-PDGF-BB with B-TCP at 61.2% and 62.0%, respectively.[7] The rate of failures, defined as delayed or nonunion requiring further surgery, was 8% in the autograft group and 7.3% in the rhPDGF-BB with B-TCP group. No anti-bodies were detected in either group at any time.[17] More recently, an injectable prep-aration has been studied. This compares a carrier of collagen and powdered B-TCP mixed with rhPDGF-BB to make in injectable slurry with autologous graft. This study demonstrated better fusion mass in the injectable group against controls. With this product licensed in Canada, a carrier of collagen and powdered B-TCP mixed with rhPDGF-BB to make in injectable slurry is almost always used in preference to the granules-alone preparation 19.

VANCOUVER INDICATIONS

With its safety and efficacy established in 3 multicenter trials, utilization of rhPDGF-BB with B-TCP has increased since its approval by Health Canada 2009 as an alternative to autograft for ankle, hindfoot, and midfoot fusions. With operating room time at a premium due to system restrictions, rh-PDGF-BB with B TCP allows for a decrease in surgical times, personnel costs, and possibly hospital length of stay when compared with autograft.

Nonunion

Determining those who are at risk of nonunion is vital in reducing the possibility of nonunion with foot and ankle surgery. Prior studies have helped in identifying the patients most at risk for this outcome and has guided usage of rh-PDGF-BB and B-TCP.[18,19] Patients who are identified to be at higher risk through use of the Nonunion Risk Assessment Model often receive either rh-PDGF-BB and B-TCP alone or as a supplement to autograft. Risk factors associated with nonunion at the authors' institution include

Tobacco use
History of nonunion
Lack of fusion site stability
Gaps at the fusion site
Poor local vascularity defined as lack of pedal pulse
Poor compliance with weight bearing
Poor soft tissue envelope
Poorly controlled diabetes
Obesity
Rheumatoid arthritis
Osteoporosis
Age older than 60
Use of nonsteroidal medications

All operative patients are screened in the clinic. If rh-PDFG-BB with B-TCP is warranted, patients are consented prior to placement.

Intraoperatively, as is standard with all arthrodesis procedures, care it taken to denude the articular cartilage and prepare the surfaces in standard fashion. Whether performed arthroscopically or open, the surfaces are opposed, and rigid internal fixation is applied. The rh-PDFG-BB and B-TCP are placed prior to rigid fixation after appropriate irrigation is applied.

Osteochondral Lesions

In addition to use in at-risk patients, the indications for rh-PDGF-BB and B-TCP has expanded. While initial treatment of osteochondral lesions consists of arthroscopic debridement and microfracture, based on recent literature from the authors' institution, rh-PDGF-BB with B-TCP shows promising results in chronic lesions without the morbidity associated with more invasive techniques.[20] In a proof-of-concept trial, 5 patients showed marked improvement in both VAS pain score and AOS functional scores. Additionally, bone healing was seen on CT, and a reduction in edema was seen on MRI.

Fusion Indications

Platelet-derived growth factor has been available in Vancouver and Canada for 10 years, either as a study device or a licensed product for foot and ankle fusions. Limitations have primarily been based on cost. Within the foot and ankle, the authors have found rh-PDGF-BB to be helpful for select patients in all areas of the foot. Currently, the injectable form of rh-PDGF-BB is used almost exclusively. The injectable form is easier to place into the fusion site, and has had excellent results with regards to union rates compared to autograft.

For segmental defects, rh-PDGF-BB has been used around iliac crest graft and femoral head allograft, in addition to internal or external fixation. These patients are at risk for nonunion, and the combination seems to be effective. For patients with diabetes and infection, fusions have been performed using a combination of rh-PDGF-BB and tobramycin carried in a calcium sulfate carrier. This assists in both resolving the infection at the site, as well as stimulating bone healing. The resolution of infection is important in assisting with fusion.

For combined ankle and subtalar fusion, an increased risk for nonunion exists. As a result, rh-PDGF-BB is routinely used in this situation at the authors' institution.

The studies performed to date did not enroll patients with nonunions, as this would be a difficult target population. However, almost all nonunions of fusions or fractures in the foot and ankle in Vancouver receive rh-PDGFBB. Cases that the authors can recollect include fracture nonunions and malunions of the distal tibia, medial or lateral malleolus, talus, calcaneus, navicular, and metatarsals. Nonunions of fusions treated include the tibiotalar joint, subtalar joint, calcaneo cuboid joint, talonavicular joint, naviculo-cuniform, tarsometatarsal, and first metatarsophalangeal joint.

Osteotomies that result in a bone gap have also been successfully treated using rh-PDGF-BB. Tibial osteotomies and lateral column lengthenings have successfully been fused using a step plate and rh-PDGF-BB in the bone deficit. It is important to remember, however, that rh-PDGF-BB is not used in primary fusions in patients who are deemed to have minimal risk of nonunion.

Growth factor is not a substitute for good surgical technique. In every case, the joint needs to be well prepared with all the cartilage removed. Cartilage contains growth factors that prevent the cytotaxis of osteoblasts, and also prevents neovascularization. Therefore residual cartilage will act against the bone graft, so complete removal will assist in the goal of achieving fusion.

Fusion site stability will also assist in achieving bony union. Fusion constructs should be carefully considered. The fusion site should be stable and should not have micro-motion. For example, plates should have a cross-screw placed, and within the authors' institution, at least 2 screws are placed across the fusion site to control the fusion site in rotation.

Since the introduction of rhPDGF-BB into the authors' practices, the rate of autogenous graft harvest has decreased considerably. The data from the injectable study and the Aminox study suggest that bone graft substitutes may result in better bone healing than autograft.[21,22] The harvest of cancellous autograft has almost ceased in high-risk patients, and graft harvest is only performed for segmental defects and usually in conjunction with the use of rh-PDGF-BB.

The reduced need for bone graft harvest has had some additional benefits. Iliac crest graft harvest was often a pivotal point in the need for admission at the authors' institution.

This has resulted in reduced admission rates and increase in daycare surgery. The authors' hospital also has an active block program and is used in conjunction with an outpatient no-sedation swing room. This requires the use of calf tourniquets and no proximal procedure. The use of rh-PDGF-BB facilitates this program, as one can avoid tibial and iliac crest grafts.

SUMMARY

The use of rh-PDGF-BB in the last 10 years has enhanced patient care and has reduced the pain, discomfort, and admission rate after surgery, and likely improved outcomes.

REFERENCES

1. DiGiovanni CW, Petricek JM. The evolution of rhPDGF-BB in musculoskeletal repair and its role in foot and ankle fusion surgery. Foot Ankle Clin 2010;15: 621–40.
2. Haddad SL, Coetzee JC, Estok R, et al. Intermediate and long-term outcomes of total ankle arthroplasty and ankle arthrodesis. A systematic review of the literature. J Bone Joint Surg Am 2007;89:1899–905.
3. Easley ME, Trnka HJ, Schon LC, et al. Isolated subtalar arthrodesis. J Bone Joint Surg Am 2000;82:613–24.
4. Krause FG, Windolf M, Bora B, et al. Impact of complications in total ankle replacement and ankle arthrodesis analyzed with a validated outcome measurement. J Bone Joint Surg Am 2011;93:830–9.
5. El-Amin SF, Hogan MV, Allen AA, et al. The indications and use of bone morphogenetic proteins in foot, ankle, and tibia surgery. Foot Ankle Clin 2010;15:543–51.
6. Solchaga LA, Hee CK, Aguiar DJ, et al. Augment bone graft products compare favorably with autologous bone graft in an ovine model of lumbar interbody spine fusion. Spine (Phila Pa 1976) 2012;37:E461–7.
7. DiGiovanni CW, Lin SS, Baumhauer JF, et al. Recombinant human platelet-derived growth factor-BB and beta-tricalcium phosphate (rhPDGF-BB/beta-TCP): an alternative to autogenous bone graft. J Bone Joint Surg Am 2013;95: 1184–92.
8. DeOrio JK, Farber DC. Morbidity associated with anterior iliac crest bone grafting in foot and ankle surgery. Foot Ankle Int 2005;26:147–51.
9. Baumhauer J, Pinzur MS, Donahue R, et al. Site selection and pain outcome after autologous bone graft harvest. Foot Ankle Int 2014;35:104–7.
10. Frohberg U, Mazock JB. A review of morbidity associated with bone harvest from the proximal tibial metaphysis. Mund Kiefer Gesichtschir 2005;9:63–5.
11. Dahlin C, Johansson A. Iliac crest autogenous bone graft versus alloplastic graft and guided bone regeneration in the reconstruction of atrophic maxillae: a 5-year retrospective study on cost-effectiveness and clinical outcome. Clin Implant Dent Relat Res 2011;13:305–10.
12. Garrison KR, Donell S, Ryder J, et al. Clinical effectiveness and cost-effectiveness of bone morphogenetic proteins in the non-healing of fractures and spinal fusion: a systematic review. Health Technol Assess 2007;11: 1–150, iii-iv.
13. Polly DW Jr, Ackerman SJ, Shaffrey CI, et al. A cost analysis of bone morphogenetic protein versus autogenous iliac crest bone graft in single-level anterior lumbar fusion. Orthopedics 2003;26:1027–37.

14. Chiodo CP, Hahne J, Wilson MG, et al. Histological differences in iliac and tibial bone graft. Foot Ankle Int 2010;31:418–22.
15. Friedlaender GE, Lin S, Solchaga LA, et al. The role of recombinant human platelet-derived growth factor-BB (rhPDGF-BB) in orthopaedic bone repair and regeneration. Curr Pharm Des 2013;19:3384–90.
16. Daniels T, DiGiovanni C, Lau JT, et al. Prospective clinical pilot trial in a single cohort group of rhPDGF in foot arthrodeses. Foot Ankle Int 2010;31:473–9.
17. Solchaga LA, Daniels T, Roach S, et al. Effect of implantation of augment((R)) bone graft on serum concentrations of platelet-derived growth factors: a pharmacokinetic study. Clin Drug Investig 2013;33:143–9.
18. Thevendran G, Wang C, Pinney SJ, et al. Nonunion risk assessment in foot and ankle surgery. proposing a predictive risk assessment model. Foot Ankle Int 2015;36:901–7.
19. Thevendran G, Younger A, Pinney S. Current concepts review: risk factors for nonunions in foot and ankle arthrodeses. Foot Ankle Int 2012;33:1031–40.
20. Younger A, Wing K, Penner M, et al. A study to evaluate the safety of platelet-derived growth factor for treatment of osteochondral defects of the talus. Knee Surg Sports Traumatol Arthrosc 2016;24:1250–8.
21. Daniels TR, Younger AS, Penner MJ, et al. Prospective randomized controlled trial of hindfoot and ankle fusions treated with rhPDGF-BB in combination with a beta-TCP-collagen matrix. Foot Ankle Int 2015;36:739–48.
22. Glazebrook M, Younger A, Wing K, et al. A prospective pilot study of B2A-coated ceramic granules (Amplex) compared to autograft for ankle and hindfoot arthrodesis. Foot Ankle Int 2013;34:1055–63.

Injectable Recombinant Human Platelet-derived Growth Factor in Collagen Carrier for Hindfoot Fusion

CrossMark

Andrew Dodd, MD, FRCSC, Timothy R. Daniels, MD, FRCSC*

KEYWORDS

• rh-PDGF • Hindfoot arthrodesis • Medial approach • Surgical technique

KEY POINTS

- Autogenous bone graft harvest is associated with significant risks and morbidity.
- Recombinant human platelet-derived growth factor is a safe, effective alternative to autogenous bone grafting in the setting of hindfoot arthrodesis.
- A single medial approach can provide adequate access to both the subtalar and talonavicular joints for double arthrodesis of the hindfoot.

INTRODUCTION

The hindfoot (minus the ankle) is composed of the talus and calcaneus, and their articulations including the subtalar joint (STJ), talonavicular joint (TNJ), and calcaneocuboid joint (CCJ). The hindfoot allows for inversion and eversion of the foot primarily through motion at the STJ and TNJ.[1,2] Its importance in normal gait lies in its ability to transform the foot from a flexible shock absorber at heel strike into a rigid lever at toe-off.[1,2] Dysfunction of the hindfoot complex may occur as a result of disease or deformity. Degenerative joint disease (inflammatory, post-traumatic, idiopathic) and/or substantial deformity can all contribute to pain and dysfunction of the hindfoot.[3–6] When nonoperative management of these problems fails, arthrodesis of 1 or more of the articulations of the hindfoot may be necessary.

Disclosures: Dr T.R. Daniels is a consultant for Wright Medical Technology. Dr A. Dodd has nothing to disclose.
Division of Orthopaedic Surgery, St. Michael's Hospital, University of Toronto, 800-55 Queen Street East, Toronto, Ontario M5C 1R6, Canada
* Corresponding author.
E-mail address: DanielsT@smh.ca

Foot Ankle Clin N Am 21 (2016) 777–791
http://dx.doi.org/10.1016/j.fcl.2016.07.013
1083-7515/16/© 2016 Elsevier Inc. All rights reserved.

In any arthrodesis procedure, nonunion (pseudoarthrosis) is a potential risk. The rate of nonunion in hindfoot fusions varies dramatically depending on the study.[3,6–12] Studies include isolated STJ fusions, double and triple fusions, and variable methods of determining union. The rate of nonunion of isolated STJ fusions may be as high as 20% and may be even higher in triple fusions.[3,6–12] Smoking has been found as a consistent risk factor for development of nonunion after hindfoot fusion procedures.[6,7] Other risk factors include poorly controlled diabetes mellitus, vasculopathy, obesity, inadequate stability at the fusion site, fusion site gaps, avascular necrosis, and noncompliance with weightbearing restrictions.[13] Rates of nonunion reported in the literature are largely based on radiographs, and this may overestimate union rates.[10] Coughlin and colleagues[10] found that radiographs consistently overestimated union rates in hindfoot fusions when compared with computed tomography scan. They also found that orthopedic surgeons tend to overestimate union rates when compared with radiologists.[10] Regardless of the true nonunion rate, symptomatic nonunion after hindfoot arthrodesis is the most common reason for revision surgery. Avoiding this complication would certainly reduce rates of reoperation.

Bone grafting to enhance healing has been used extensively for decades. Although no consensus exists on the necessity of bone grafting, surgeons must take into account many factors when making the decision to use any type of bone graft material. Both clinical and radiographic factors play a role. Common reasons for the use of bone graft include nonunion surgery, history of nonunion at other sites, smoking, diabetes, renal disease, osteonecrosis, bone loss, and significant deformity.[14] Autogenous iliac crest bone graft has historically been the most common source for bone graft material.[15–17] Other sources for autogenous bone graft material have also been extensively reported included the proximal and distal tibia, greater trochanter, and calcaneus.[15] Each of these sites has their own risks associated with bone harvest, with common complications including pain, infection, and nerve injury.[12,15–19] Synthetic alternatives to autogenous bone graft offer an alternative method of enhancing bone growth while preventing the potential morbidity of bone graft harvest.[17]

Platelet-derived growth factor (PDGF) is a cytokine secreted by platelets and cells of mesenchymal origin at the site of fracture and soft tissue injury.[20–22] This growth factor acts as a chemotactic and mitogenic agent, attracting mesenchymal cells to the area of injury, and inducing replication and differentiation into osteogenic cells.[20–23] In addition, PDGF is proangiogenic, resulting in increased blood flow to the area of injury.[20–22] Recombinant human PDGF (rhPDGF-BB) is a subtype of PDGF synthesized for use in research and clinical settings. Numerous animal and basic science studies have demonstrated the efficacy and safety of PDGF and rhPDGF-BB for use in bone and soft tissue healing.[20–22]

Recent clinical studies examining the efficacy of rhPDGF in patients undergoing ankle and hindfoot fusions have demonstrated at least equivalent fusion rates when compared with cancellous autograft.[24,25] Data from a large Canadian randomized controlled trial suggest that fusion rates may even be greater for rhPDGF delivered in a collagen-based matrix than for autograft.[24] These clinical studies have also further validated the safety of using PDGF in foot and ankle surgery.

INDICATIONS AND CONTRAINDICATIONS

Indications for rh-PDGF can be grouped as disease- and patient-specific factors that increase the risk of nonunion (**Box 1**). Contraindications are few and most are related to clinical situations in which the safety of rhPDGF is unknown (**Box 2**).

Box 1
Indications for use of platelet-derived growth factor

Patient Specific

Current or past smoker

Nonunion/pseudoarthrosis

Significant deformity correction

History of impaired bone healing

Bone loss

Disease Specific

Diabetes mellitus type 1 or 2

Vasculopathy

Immunosuppression (disease or medications)

SURGICAL TECHNIQUE: DOUBLE ARTHRODESIS THROUGH A MEDIAL APPROACH (TALONAVICULAR/SUBTALAR JOINTS)
Preoperative Planning

History

A thorough medical and surgical history is necessary to elucidate risk factors for nonunion and other complications. Important information to document includes the following:

- Previous surgical procedures
  - Type of procedures
  - Intraoperative and postoperative complications
  - Infections
- Diabetic patients
  - Insulin dependent or noninsulin dependent
  - Diabetic control (hemoglobin A1C levels)

Box 2
Contraindications to the use of rh-PDGF

Contraindications

Allergy to product/product components

Inadequate soft tissue coverage[a]

Safety Unknown

Active infection

Active or history of cancer

Pregnancy/breastfeeding

Metabolic bone disease (other than osteoporosis/diabetes mellitus)

Pediatric patients (<18 years of age or open physes)

Prior use of rhPDGF

Abbreviation: rhPDGF, recombinant human platelet-derived growth factor.
  [a] Contraindication to both use of PDGF and to ankle fusion.

- o Presence of neuropathy, retinopathy, nephropathy
- o History of nonhealing wounds
- Smoking status
  - o Current or former smoker
  - o Number of pack-years smoked
- Vasculopathy
  - o Cardiac or peripheral vascular disease
- Metabolic bone disease
  - o Type and severity
- Medications
  - o Anticoagulants
  - o Bone-healing inhibitors (nonsteroidal antiinflammatory drugs)

Physical examination

A comprehensive physical examination of the affected extremity should focus on the following.

- Deformity
  - o Degree
  - o Planes of deformity
  - o Flexibility
  - o Adjacent joint deformity (knee, ankle, forefoot)
  - o Soft tissue contractures
- Soft tissue envelope
  - o Integrity of soft tissues
  - o Surgical scars
  - o Signs of vascular insufficiency
- Neurovascular status
  - o Sensation
  - o Motor function
  - o Presence or absence of pulses

Diagnostic imaging

All patients should have weight bearing radiographs, including a complete foot and ankle series (standing anteroposterior/lateral views of the foot and ankle, hindfoot alignment view).[4,5,26] Computed tomography scans (weight bearing or non–weight bearing) may be included in cases with significant deformity and/or to assess the degree of involvement of adjacent joints and bone stock. Other imaging studies may be included in patient-specific situations (**Table 1**).

Patient Preparation and Positioning

The patient is positioned supine on a radiolucent operating room table. The resting position of the limb is typically in external rotation, which is ideal for the medial approach to the hindfoot. A pneumatic tourniquet is placed as proximal on the thigh as possible and set to 300 mm Hg. The limb is prepared and draped above the knee to assist with foot positioning intraoperatively. Ensure the limb is accessible for intraoperative fluoroscopy.

Surgical Approach

The order of preparation of the joints is influenced by the deformity and the degree of arthritis and/or contracture. In most circumstances, the senior author prefers to prepare the TNJ first, followed by the STJ. The decision to fuse the CCJ is left until

Table 1
Diagnostic imaging studies to consider preoperatively

Study	When to Consider	Important Results
Weight bearing radiographs	All patients	Arthropathy, deformity, bone stock
CT scan	Questionable bone stock Severe deformity Avascular necrosis	Adjacent joint disease, deformity, bone stock
MRI	Possible osteomyelitis or associated soft tissue pathology Osteochondral defects Avascular necrosis	Presence of infection, vascularity of talus
Doppler ultrasound or CT angiography	Abnormal vascular examination	Reversible/treatable vascular disease

Abbreviation: CT, computed tomography.

assessment of deformity correction is made after adequate preparation and provisional fixation of the STJ and TNJ. If the CCJ is arthritic, then it is fused regardless of the deformity correction required. If this is the case, then the CCJ and STJ are prepared via a sinus tarsi approach.

1. Make the skin incision (**Fig. 1**).
   a. The skin incision is between the tibialis anterior and posterior tibial tendon (PTT), on the medial border of the foot. The incision is performed closer to the PTT, inferior to the midline between the tibialis anterior tendon and the PTT.
   b. Begin proximally at the medial malleolus and extend distally several centimeters past the navicular tuberosity (~8 cm incision).
   c. Develop full-thickness fasciocutaneous flaps superior and inferior.
2. Open the PTT sheath (**Fig. 2**).
   a. Palpate inferiorly to find the tendon sheath of the PTT.
   b. Incise sharply along the course of the tendon sheath, freeing up the tendon.
   c. In cases of a degenerative or insufficient tendon, the tendon may be excised.
   d. If the tendon is healthy, it may be retracted inferiorly as necessary.
3. Open the TNJ capsule (**Fig. 3**).
   a. Palpate the TNJ, just proximal to the navicular tuberosity.
   b. Use fluoroscopy to localize the joint if it is not easily identified.

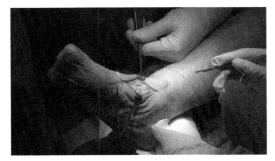

Fig. 1. Skin incision.

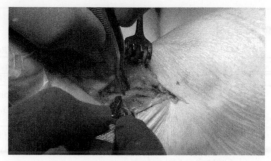

Fig. 2. Opening of the posterior tibial tendon sheath (in forceps).

    c. Incise the TNJ capsule in line with the skin incision and elevate flaps superiorly and inferiorly.

    d. The PTT is reflected off of the navicular tuberosity. This plantar dissection can be extended distally, past the medial naviculocuneiform joint to aid in exposing the inferior aspect of the TNJ.

    e. Expose the TNJ enough to ensure adequate visualization for debridement, but minimize dissection off the dorsal aspect of the talar neck to preserve the dorsal vascular ring. This step is particularly important in severe pes planus deformities where the artery of the sinus tarsi is often compromised by chronic impingement. Avascular necrosis of the anterolateral portion of the talar body has been reported in double fusions via a medial approach.[27–29]

4. Expose the STJ (**Fig. 4**).

    a. Exposure of the STJ medially uses the interval between the talar neck and the anterior/middle facets of the calcaneus.

    b. Retract the PTT and spring ligament inferiorly.

    c. Dissect inferiorly along the talar neck, along the anterior/middle facets. Removing cartilage from this area helps to increase the working space and create an area where a laminar spreader can be inserted. External pin-distractors are also useful in exposing the STJ.

    d. A readily visible landmark for the STJ is the sustentaculum tali, which can be palpated inferior to the medial malleolus when the PTT is resected or retracted inferiorly.

    e. Mobilize tissue from the medial calcaneal body to enhance exposure of the STJ. Take care not to disrupt the deltoid ligament insertion to the talar body, because this can disrupt the deltoid artery and talar body blood supply.

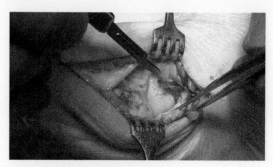

Fig. 3. Exposure of the talonavicular joint.

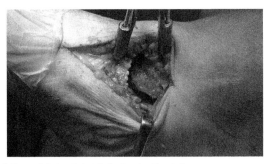

Fig. 4. Exposure of the subtalar joint inferior to the talus.

Surgical Procedure

Step 1: Prepare the TNJ (**Fig. 5**).

- Insert a laminar spreader or pin-distractor to open the joint and allow adequate debridement. If a laminar spreader is used, avoid the plantar half of the joint because the talar bone is soft and this can lead to impaction of the talar head. Place the laminar spreader on the dorsolateral aspect of the joint where the best bone is present.
- The talar head is often very soft in the medial and plantar aspects; remove cartilage from the plantarmedial aspect of the talar head first. Often a rongeur is sufficient. This helps to open up the TNJ. If a laminar spreader is used, it is best located in the dorsolateral aspects of the joint where the bone is harder and will not impact with distraction forces. In pes planus deformities the anterolateral aspect of the TNJ can be difficult to access. The surgeon will have to make a special effort to expose and debride the anterolateral aspect of the TNJ, which often means working around the talar head and debriding areas by feel, without direct visualization. In addition, a large talar beak is often present on the anterolateral border of the talar head/neck junction. This can be removed from either the medial incision or a separate sinus tarsi incision if deemed necessary.
- Debride all remaining articular cartilage with a combination of sharp osteotomes, curettes, and rongeurs.
- A power burr is used to remove eburnated subchondral bone and expose cancellous bone.
  - Remove only as much bone as is necessary to expose cancellous bone while maximizing remaining bone stock for the fusion mass.

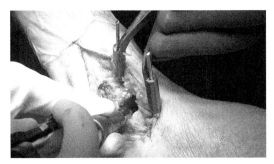

Fig. 5. Talonavicular joint preparation. A pin-distractor is used to open the joint and a power burr aids with debridement.

- Last, a 2.0-mm drill is used to drill the talar and navicular bone surfaces to enhance vascular inflow to the fusion site
- In pes planus deformities, a shortening of the medial column is required and is often achieved by normal debridement of the joint. After reduction there is often gapping at the lateral aspect of the TNJ, most appreciated on the anteroposterior fluoroscopic view of the foot. This void should be filled with bone graft.
- In pes cavus deformities, lengthening of the medial column is required. In severe deformities, good bone-on-bone apposition at the TNJ area may only be achieved by performing a resection arthrodesis of the CCJ, thus effectively shortening the lateral column and improving apposition of the navicular on the talar head. If gapping continues on the medial aspect of the TNJ, this area should be filled with bone graft.

Step 2: Prepare the STJ (**Fig. 6**).

- Clear the sinus tarsi of soft tissue; this improves visualization of the posterior facet. The posterior facet at this level is best engaged by working in a superior direction using the anterior inferior portion of the talar body as a reference point.
- Remove the remaining cartilage and debride the anterior aspect of the STJ in preparation for inserting a laminar spreader or application of pin-distractor. As cartilage is removed, the posterior facet becomes more visible and the space available to insert a laminar spreader becomes larger.
- If using a laminar spreader initially, place it in the anterior aspect of the posterior facet, near the interosseous ligament, and debride the lateral aspect of the posterior facet first.
- Once the lateral aspect of posterior facet has been prepared, insert the laminar spreader along the lateral border of the posterior facet and prepare the medial aspect of the joint. This will also allow access to the anterior and middle facets of the STJ.
- Medial dissection should proceed until the flexor hallucis longus tendon is visualized to ensure adequate preparation of the posteromedial joint. Medial exposure of the posterior facet can be difficult and takes careful dissection and time.
- A power burr is used to remove eburnated subchondral bone and expose cancellous bone.
  - Remove only as much bone as is necessary to expose cancellous bone while maximizing remaining bone stock for the fusion mass.
- Last, a 2.0-mm drill is used to drill the talar and calcaneal bone surfaces to enhance vascular inflow to the fusion site.

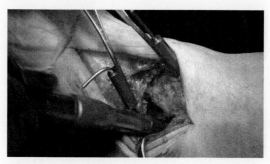

Fig. 6. Preparation of the subtalar joint. A burr is inserted into the subtalar joint as part of joint preparation.

- Ensure that the entire posterior facet of the STJ has been adequately debrided on both the talar and calcaneal surfaces.
  - The posteromedial corner is an area that is commonly inadequately debrided, because this area is not easily visualized.
- Proper positioning of the calcaneus under the talus is only possible when an adequate debridement of the STJ has been performed. In cases that require a TNJ fusion owing to deformity and/or arthritis, the TNJ will require adequate debridement and release before the calcaneus can be rotated and repositioned under the talus. The surgeon should aim to have the STJ reduced in a neutral or slightly externally rotated position, which will naturally place the calcaneus in slight valgus. Placing the calcaneus in a slight valgus is achieved with slight external rotation of the calcaneus; attaining this position is not through a hinging (abduction) motion as depicted in some textbooks.

Step 3: Calcaneus guidewire placement (**Fig. 7**).

- A guidewire from a 6.5-, 7.0-, or 7.3-mm cannulated screw system is inserted from the posterior aspect of the calcaneal tuberosity just proximal to the weight bearing surface
- The wires are advanced through the central portion of the posterior facet of the STJ in the trajectory of the talar body/neck area. The endpoint of the guidewire is toward the anterior and medial aspect of the talar neck/head area (see **Fig. 7**A).
- Distracting the joint allows confirmation of the position of the wire in the posterior facet of the STJ.
- Confirm acceptable wire positioning on fluoroscopy.
- Leave the wire flush with the calcaneal surface of the STJ until appropriate positioning of the joints.
- A second guidewire can be placed from the anterior aspect of the calcaneus into the talar neck/body junction. The starting point is approximately 1 cm from the CCJ at an angle perpendicular to the talar neck (see **Fig. 7**B).

Step 4: Navicular guidewire placement (**Fig. 8**).

- A guidewire for a 4.5-mm cannulated screw is inserted into the navicular, starting at the plantar–medial aspect of the navicular tuberosity.
- It is advanced in a dorsal–lateral direction toward the talar head.
- Distracting the joint allows confirmation of a central exit point in the TNJ.
- Confirm acceptable wire positioning on fluoroscopy.

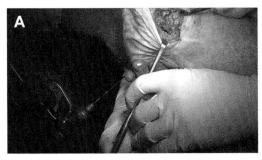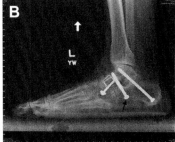

Fig. 7. (*A*) Insertion of guidewire for subtalar joint fixation with a cannulated screw. (*B*) Example of a second screw used to stabilize the subtalar joint (*arrow*). The screw is placed from plantarlateral in the calcaneus to dorsomedial in the talar head/neck.

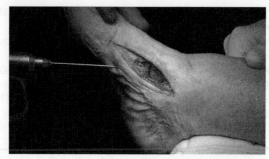

Fig. 8. Insertion of talonavicular joint guidewire for cannulated screw.

- Leave the wire flush with the proximal navicular surface until appropriate positioning of the joints.

Step 5: Injection of rhPDGF (**Fig. 9**).

- Final irrigation of the joints is performed.
- The rhPDGF is injected into the talonavicular and STJ fusion sites.
- Avoid the use of irrigation after injection.

Step 6: Advancement of guidewires (**Fig. 10**).

- The foot is positioned into the position desired for fusion. The senior author prefers to externally rotate the calcaneus into the desired position first. The surgeon can use the anterolateral aspect of the talar body as a guide; it should align with the corresponding anterolateral aspect of the posterior facet on the calcaneus. The small finger of the surgeon can often be inserted comfortably in the sinus tarsi area after the calcaneus is properly positioned.
- Advance the subtalar guidewire into the talus.
- Use fluoroscopy liberally to ensure safe positioning of the wires without penetration into the ankle joint.
- Once the calcaneus is provisionally stabilized in the desired position, attention is turned to the TNJ. The midfoot/forefoot is rotated into a neutral position (from a pronated position in pes planus deformities and a supinated position in forefoot-driven cavovarus deformities). In pes planus deformities, a Dewar or Cobb is placed under the talar neck and a superiorly directed force is applied to elevate the talar neck. The navicular is then translated dorsally to help reduce the plantarly subluxed navicular to the talar head.

Step 7: Placement of cannulated screws (**Fig. 11**).

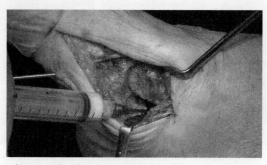

Fig. 9. Recombinant human platelet-derived growth factor injection into the subtalar joint and talonavicular joint.

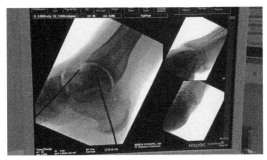

Fig. 10. Reduction and temporary stabilization of the subtalar joint and talonavicular joint has been performed and is checked fluoroscopically.

- The talonavicular guidewire is overdrilled with a cannulated 3.2-mm drill.
- A partially threaded 4.5-mm cannulated screw of appropriate depth is inserted (with or without a washer as necessary).
- The subtalar guidewires are overdrilled with a 4.5-mm cannulated drill.
- A 7.3-mm partially threaded cannulated screw is inserted to compress the STJ fusion site.

Step 8: Additional talonavicular fixation (**Figs. 12** and **13**).

- Additional fixation of the TNJ is added as necessary.
- Options include staples, plate/screw constructs, or additional cannulated screws. Under fluoroscopic guidance, an additional screw can be placed percutaneously from the anterolateral aspect of the navicular into the talar head/neck, which will aid in compression of the lateral aspect of the TNJ.

Step 9: Closure and Splinting.

- Before closure, final fluoroscopic images are taken to ensure acceptable position of the joints and hardware.

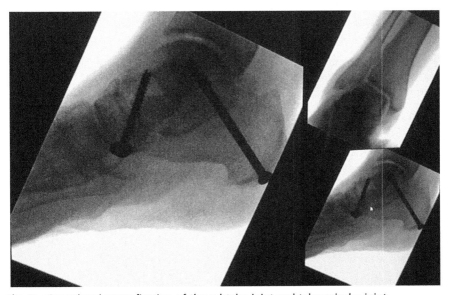

Fig. 11. Cannulated screw fixation of the subtalar joint and talonavicular joint.

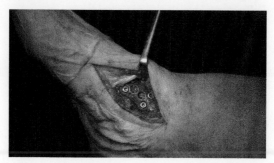

Fig. 12. Additional plate fixation of the talonavicular joint has been performed.

- The goal is a watertight deep closure to contain the rh-PDGF before deflating the tourniquet.
- Deep fascia is closed with a 1-0 Vicryl suture.
- Subcutaneous tissue is closed with interrupted, inverted 2-0 Vicryl suture.
- Skin is closed with 3-0 running subcuticular monofilament.
- A sterile dressing is applied.
- A well-padded posterior slab with stirrup is applied to hold the foot in a plantigrade position.

Complications and Management

Complications can range from superficial surgical site infection to deep infection and nonunion. Management should be tailored to the clinical situation. General principles are outlined in **Table 2**.

Postoperative Care

The typical postoperative course is described in **Table 3**. Any complications that arise may change this plan as described.

Outcomes

Historical rates of nonunion in hindfoot fusions have been high.[6,9–11,22] Synthesizing data is challenging owing to the heterogeneity in arthritis etiology, patient

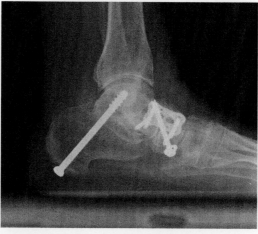

Fig. 13. Postoperative radiograph of a double arthrodesis.

Table 2
General principles of complications and management

Complication	Management
Superficial wound infection	Oral antibiotics
Delayed wound healing/dehiscence	Local wound care Close follow-up With or without oral antibiotics With or without surgical debridement and revision closure
Deep infection	Surgical debridement IV antibiotics
Delayed/nonunion	CT scan: confirm diagnosis Nonpainful: no intervention Painful: consider revision fusion
Broken hardware	Nonpainful: no intervention Painful: consider CT scan to assess union
Malunion	Revision surgery at discretion of surgeon

Abbreviations: CT, computed tomography; IV, intravenous.

comorbidities, and surgical/fixation techniques. Recent studies examining union rates after double arthrodesis through a single medial incision demonstrate high union rates.[30–32] It should be noted, however, that these articles do not report on risk factors for nonunion, and that orthobiologics were used in many cases to stimulate union.

Clinical results of hindfoot fusion with rhPDGF demonstrate high overall union rates.[24,25] Union rates in high-risk patients are at least equivalent with rhPDGF-BB in combination with a beta-tricalcium phosphate–collagen matrix when compared with cancellous autograft.[24] In a large randomized controlled trial, a fusion rate of 86.4% was found with rhPDGF-BB (81 joints) compared with 67.0% for cancellous autograft (230 joints) as determined by computed tomography scan at 24 weeks postoperatively.

Although many factors affect clinical outcomes, union has a substantial impact. Patient outcomes after nonunion are inferior compared with union.[8] Glazebrook and

Table 3
A typical postoperative course

No. of Weeks Postoperative	Plan
2	Remove postoperative splint Wound check Apply fiberglass cast Non–weight bearing
6	Remove fiberglass cast Initiate range of motion exercises Apply removable cast-boot Bear weight as tolerated in cast-boot
12	Remove cast-boot Initiate weight bearing as tolerated Initiate rehabilitation/physiotherapy as needed Gradually return to activities as tolerated
24	Final radiographs to confirm fusion

colleagues[33] have demonstrated that patient outcomes are directly related to the degree of osseous bridging in patients undergoing hindfoot fusion. The use of rhPDGF to enhance union rates should be considered in high-risk patients to maximize patient outcome and minimize the need for revision surgery.

SUMMARY

The addition of rhPDGF to hindfoot fusion in patients at high risk for nonunion is safe and effective. Union rates are comparable with autogenous iliac crest bone graft with significantly lower morbidity. No modification of surgical technique is necessary when using rhPDGF and a separate bone harvesting procedure is avoided. Double arthrodesis through a single medial approach demonstrates high union rates in the literature, and the addition of rhPDGF can be expected to enhance union rates in high-risk patients.

REFERENCES

1. Maceira E, Monteagudo M. Subtalar anatomy and mechanics. Foot Ankle Clin 2015;20(2):195–221.
2. Coughlin MJ, Mann RA, Saltzman CL. Surgery of the Foot and Ankle. Philadelphia, PA: Mosby Elsevier; 2007. p. 1467–8.
3. Pell RF, Myerson MS, Schon LC. Clinical outcome after primary triple arthrodesis. J Bone Joint Surg Am 2000;82(1):47–57.
4. Greisberg J, Sangeorzan B. Hindfoot arthrodesis. J Am Acad Orthop Surg 2007; 15(1):65–71.
5. Wapner KL. Triple arthrodesis in adults. J Am Acad Orthop Surg 1998;6(3): 188–96.
6. Easley ME, Trnka HJ, Schon LC, et al. Isolated subtalar arthrodesis. J Bone Joint Surg Am 2000;82(5):613–24.
7. Ishikawa SN, Murphy GA, Richardson EG. The effect of cigarette smoking on hindfoot fusions. Foot Ankle Int 2002;23(11):996–8.
8. Davies MB, Rosenfeld PF, Stavrou P, et al. A comprehensive review of subtalar arthrodesis. Foot Ankle Int 2007;28(3):295–7.
9. de Groot IB, Reijman M, Luning HA, et al. Long-term results after a triple arthrodesis of the hindfoot: function and satisfaction in 36 patients. Int Orthop 2008; 32(2):237–41.
10. Coughlin MJ, Grimes JS, Traughber PD, et al. Comparison of radiographs and CT scans in the prospective evaluation of the fusion of hindfoot arthrodesis. Foot Ankle Int 2006;27(10):780–7.
11. Angus PD, Cowell HR. Triple arthrodesis. A critical long-term review. J Bone Joint Surg Br 1986;68(2):260–5.
12. DiGiovanni CW, Lin SS, Baumhauer JF, et al. Recombinant human platelet-derived growth factor-BB and beta-tricalcium phosphate (rhPDGF-BB/beta-TCP): an alternative to autogenous bone graft. J Bone Joint Surg Am 2013; 95(13):1184–92.
13. Thevendran G, Wang C, Pinney SJ, et al. Nonunion risk assessment in foot and ankle surgery: proposing a predictive risk assessment model. Foot Ankle Int 2015;36(8):901–7.
14. Baumhauer JF, Pinzur MS, Daniels TR, et al. Survey on the need for bone graft in foot and ankle fusion surgery. Foot Ankle Int 2013;34(12):1629–33.
15. Fitzgibbons TC, Hawks MA, McMullen ST, et al. Bone grafting in surgery about the foot and ankle: indications and techniques. J Am Acad Orthop Surg 2011; 19(2):112–20.

16. DeOrio JK, Farber DC. Morbidity associated with anterior iliac crest bone grafting in foot and ankle surgery. Foot Ankle Int 2005;26(2):147–51.

17. Scranton PE Jr. Use of bone graft substitutes in lower extremity reconstructive surgery. Foot Ankle Int 2002;23(8):689–92.

18. Chou LB, Mann RA, Coughlin MJ, et al. Stress fracture as a complication of autogenous bone graft harvest from the distal tibia. Foot Ankle Int 2007;28(2): 199–201.

19. Loeffler BJ, Kellam JF, Sims SH, et al. Prospective observational study of donor-site morbidity following anterior iliac crest bone-grafting in orthopaedic trauma reconstruction patients. J Bone Joint Surg Am 2012;94(18):1649–54.

20. Hollinger JO, Hart CE, Hirsch SN, et al. Recombinant human platelet-derived growth factor: biology and clinical applications. J Bone Joint Surg Am 2008; 90(Suppl 1):48–54.

21. Solchaga LA, Hee CK, Roach S, et al. Safety of recombinant human platelet-derived growth factor-BB in Augment((R)) Bone Graft. J Tissue Eng 2012;3(1). 2041731412442668.

22. DiGiovanni CW, Petricek JM. The evolution of rhPDGF-BB in musculoskeletal repair and its role in foot and ankle fusion surgery. Foot Ankle Clin 2010;15(4): 621–40.

23. Lieberman JR, Daluiski A, Einhorn TA. The role of growth factors in the repair of bone. Biology and clinical applications. J Bone Joint Surg Am 2002;84-A(6): 1032–44.

24. Daniels TR, Younger AS, Penner MJ, et al. Prospective randomized controlled trial of hindfoot and ankle fusions treated with rhPDGF-BB in combination with a beta-TCP-collagen matrix. Foot Ankle Int 2015;36(7):739–48.

25. Digiovanni CW, Baumhauer J, Lin SS, et al. Prospective, randomized, multi-center feasibility trial of rhPDGF-BB versus autologous bone graft in a foot and ankle fusion model. Foot Ankle Int 2011;32(4):344–54.

26. Saltzman CL, el-Khoury GY. The hindfoot alignment view. Foot Ankle Int 1995; 16(9):572–6.

27. Galli MM, Scott RT, Bussewitz B, et al. Structures at risk with medial double hind-foot fusion: a cadaveric study. J Foot Ankle Surg 2014;53(5):598–600.

28. Phisitkul P, Haugsdal J, Vaseenon T, et al. Vascular disruption of the talus: comparison of two approaches for triple arthrodesis. Foot Ankle Int 2013;34(4): 568–74.

29. Rohm J, Zwicky L, Horn Lang T, et al. Mid- to long-term outcome of 96 corrective hindfoot fusions in 84 patients with rigid flatfoot deformity. Bone Joint J 2015; 97-B(5):668–74.

30. Anand P, Nunley JA, DeOrio JK. Single-incision medial approach for double arthrodesis of hindfoot in posterior tibialis tendon dysfunction. Foot Ankle Int 2013;34(3):338–44.

31. Knupp M, Schuh R, Stufkens SA, et al. Subtalar and talonavicular arthrodesis through a single medial approach for the correction of severe planovalgus deformity. J Bone Joint Surg Br 2009;91(5):612–5.

32. Weinraub GM, Schuberth JM, Lee M, et al. Isolated medial incisional approach to subtalar and talonavicular arthrodesis. J Foot Ankle Surg 2010;49(4):326–30.

33. Glazebrook M, Beasley W, Daniels T, et al. Establishing the relationship between clinical outcome and extent of osseous bridging between computed tomography assessment in isolated hindfoot and ankle fusions. Foot Ankle Int 2013;34(12): 1612–8.

Role of Recombinant Human Bone Morphogenetic Protein-2 on Hindfoot Arthrodesis

Jeremy Hreha, MD[a], Ethan S. Krell, MBS[a,1],
Christopher Bibbo, DO, DPM, FACS[b],*

KEYWORDS

- rhBMP-2 • Hindfoot • Arthrodesis • Fusion • Orthobiologics

KEY POINTS

- Despite improvements in fixation technique, hindfoot arthrodesis continues to be associated with modest nonunion rates.
- Of commercially available recombinant human bone morphogenetic proteins (rhBMPs), rhBMP-2 has the most osteogenic activity.
- The only study investigating the use of rhBMP-2 in hindfoot arthrodesis found a statistically significant increase in fusion rate compared with controls.
- rhBMP-2 is a valid treatment option for hindfoot arthrodesis.

INTRODUCTION

Despite advances in surgical technique, the treatment of hindfoot arthrodesis continues to be associated with complications, including delayed union, malunion, and nonunion.[1] Nonunion rates have been reported as high as 20% for triple arthrodesis.[2,3] Clain and Baxter[4] in 1994 demonstrated a nonunion rate of 6.25% for simultaneous calcaneocuboid and talonavicular fusions. Furthermore, the nonunion rates for isolated subtalar fusion, isolated talonavicular fusion and isolated calcaneocuboid fusion have been reported up to 16%,[5–11] 35%,[12–15] and 20%,[16] respectively.

Disclosure Statement: The authors have nothing to disclose.
[a] Department of Orthopaedics, Rutgers New Jersey Medical School, 185 South Orange Avenue, Newark, NJ 07103, USA; [b] Department of Orthopaedics, The Rubin Institute for Advanced Orthopaedics at Sinai Hospital, 2401 West Belvedere Avenue, Baltimore, MD 21215, USA
[1] Present address: 10 Barchester Way, Westfield, NJ 07090.
* Corresponding author.
E-mail address: drchrisbibbo@gmail.com

In addition, there can be many contributing factors associated with poor bone healing, including diabetes mellitus, smoking, immunosuppression, multiple surgeries, infection, rheumatoid arthritis, and pharmaceutical agents.[17–23] Chahal and colleagues[19] in 2006 reported that diabetic patients were 18.7 times more likely to develop malunion after isolated subtalar arthrodesis and Ishikawa and colleagues[20] in 2002 determined that smokers have a 2.7 times greater risk of developing a nonunion in hindfoot fusions compared with nonsmokers. In addition, the rate of union is significantly decreased by the failure of a previous subtalar arthrodesis.[5]

Improvements in fixation techniques and the use of bone grafts have been introduced to reduce nonunion rates. Autogenous bone graft has been beneficial in hindfoot arthrodesis enhancement owing to its intrinsic osteogenic and osteoinductive properties.[24] However, autogenous bone graft has potential limitations. The patient's age and size may restrict the quality and volume of autogenous bone graft obtainable. In addition, harvesting iliac crest bone can yield numerous minor complications, including acute and chronic donor site pain, gait disturbances, stress fractures, paraesthesias, and superficial infections, as well as major complications, including pelvic fracture, arterial injury, hernia, and peritoneal perforation.[25]

As an alternative to autologous iliac bone graft, adjuvant osteobiologics are being used in foot and ankle surgery. Osteobiologics are subcomponents of living cells that enhance the healing potential of bone via osteoinduction, osteoconduction, or osteogenesis. The osteobiologics used in foot and ankle surgery include platelet rich plasma, recombinant human platelet-derived growth factor, recombinant human bone morphogenetic proteins (rhBMPs) and bone marrow concentrate.[26] This paper investigates the role of rhBMPs, specifically rhBMP-2, in hindfoot arthrodesis.

BONE MORPHOGENETIC PROTEINS

Bone morphogenetic proteins (BMPs) were first reported in the literature by Urist in 1965[27] and more than 20 BMPs have been subsequently identified.[28] BMPs belong to the transforming growth factor superfamily and have chondroinductive and osteoinductive activity.[29] BMPs are composed of 2 major glycosylated subunits that are linked together by a disulfide bond. BMPs interact with 2 of 6 known surface receptors and initiate signal transduction via serine/threonine kinase receptors.[30,31] Activation of these intrinsic receptor serine/threonine kinases phosphorylates SMAD proteins that translocate into the nucleus leading to the expression of osteogenic-specific genes.[31,32] In addition, an alternate mechanism involves the mitogen-activated protein kinase pathway leading to the activation of p38.[31] Recent data suggest involvement of the RAS pathway and Erk kinase pathway, yet additional research into the regulation of these pathways and receptors are needed.[31,33,34] As with all signaling cascades, the BMP signaling pathway is highly regulated. Noggin, inhibin, and BMP-3 have been identified as BMP receptor antagonists[35,36] and additional proteins can block the action of the SMADs.[37] The availability of endogenous BMP is also regulated sclerostin, chordin, connective tissue growth factor (CTGF), follistatin, and gremlin regulate BMP availability.[36] Furthermore, BMP-2 has been determined to induce osteoblast differentiation of mesenchymal stem cells.[38]

BONE MORPHOGENETIC PROTEINS IN ANIMAL MODELS

BMPs play an important role locally at the fracture callus during bone healing. Bostrom and colleagues[39] in 1995 reported expression of BMP-2 and BMP-4 within the fracture callus after the fracture of rat femurs. Rabbit model studies have revealed that after administration, rhBMP-2 will stay locally at the fracture site for approximately

2 weeks.[40] Furthermore, there have been numerous animal model studies that have shown the osteoinductive potential of BMPs.[41–46] Both BMP-2 and BMP-7 have been shown to result in radiographic union in rat segmental defect models.[41–44] Similarly, Gerhart and colleagues[45] 1993 reported a 100% union rate (n = 6) and increased bending strength after rhBMP-2 treatment to a 2.5-cm segmental defect in a sheep femur. In closed tibial fractures created in skeletally mature goats, treatment with rhBMP-2 in an absorbable collagen sponge resulted in improved radiographic healing scores and biomechanical properties at 6 weeks compared with fracture controls.[46]

BONE MORPHOGENETIC PROTEINS IN CLINICAL USE

In an attempt to augment the bone-healing response, 2 rhBMPs have become commercially available: rhBMP-2 (INFUSE, Medtronic, Minneapolis, MN) and rhBMP-7 (OP-1, Stryker, Kalamazoo, MI). When compared, rhBMP-2 was determined to have more osteogenic activity than rhBMP-7.[38] Presently, rhBMP-2 has received approval from the US Food and Drug Administration for use in interbody spine fusion, acute tibial fractures, and maxillofacial bone grafting produces[47] and continues to be used for many off-label uses particularly in foot and ankle surgery.[48] There is very little literature about the efficacy of rhBMP-2 in foot and ankle surgical procedures and the indications for the application of rhBMP-2 in hindfoot arthrodesis has yet to be defined.

RECOMBINANT HUMAN BONE MORPHOGENETIC PROTEIN-2 IN HINDFOOT ARTHRODESIS

To date, only 1 study has specifically examined the use of rhBMP-2 in hindfoot arthrodesis, yet there is evidence of their effectiveness. Bibbo and colleagues[49] in 2009 reported a significant increase in fusion rates after adjuvant rhBMP-2 at 12 weeks after surgery compared with historical data (96% in rhBMP-2 treated fusions vs 48% in fusion alone). In addition, they investigated the fusion rates of each of the 3 hindfoot joints.

For isolated subtalar fusions, a total of 41 subtalar fusions were performed using rhBMP-2 with an overall union rate of 95%.[49] Among the 39 successful fusions, 27 were treated with rhBMP-2 alone and healed at a mean time of 10.4 weeks (median, 10). In addition, 8 healed after autograft and rhBMP-2 at a mean time of 13.2 weeks and 6 healed after allograft and rhBMP-2 at a mean time of 19.2 weeks. Time to union between the groups was not statistically significant.

For isolated talonavicular fusions using only rhBMP-2, a 95% union rate in 19 was reported with a mean time to union of 12.7 weeks (median, 10).[49] For isolated calcaneocuboid fusions using rhBMP-2, a total of 20 calcaneocuboid fusions were performed with an overall union rate of 95%.[49] Among the 20 successful fusions, 14 were treated with rhBMP-2 alone and healed at a mean time of 11 weeks (median, 12). In addition, 1 healed after autograft and rhBMP-2 at a mean time of 12 weeks (median, 12) and 4 healed after allograft and rhBMP-2 at a mean time of 10.2 weeks (median, 12). There was no difference in time to union between the groups.

RECOMBINANT HUMAN BONE MORPHOGENETIC PROTEIN-2 IN ANKLE ARTHRODESIS

Literature on the use of rhBMP-2 in ankle arthrodesis remains sparse; however, there is evidence of promising results. A retrospective review of 82 ankle fusions treated with rhBMP-2 showed that patients were more likely to achieve fusion (93% vs 53%) and obtained more bone bridging on computed tomography scans (48% vs

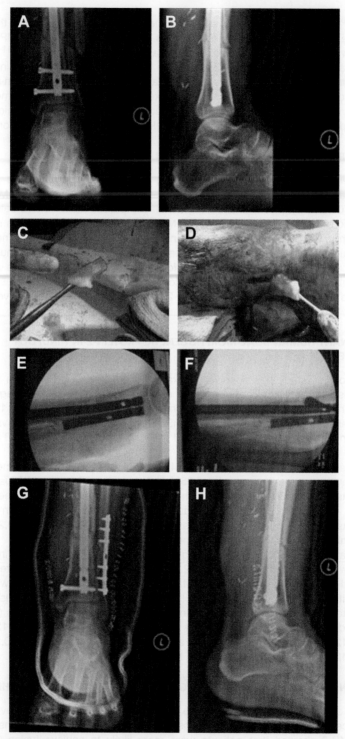

Fig. 1. A 36-year-old man who underwent open reduction and internal fixation of a left open distal tibia–fibula fracture with a free flap. The patient presented with a malunion/

32%).[50] In high-risk patients, similar results are reported. Bibbo and colleagues[49] in 2009 reported a 100% union rate in 24 high-risk ankle fusions treated with rhBMP-2 and reported fusion at a mean of 9.1 weeks (median, 8).

RECOMBINANT HUMAN BONE MORPHOGENETIC PROTEIN-2 IN TIBIOTALOCALCANEAL ARTHRODESIS

Additional exploration of the role of rhBMP-2 in tibiotalocalcaneal arthrodesis is needed; there is only 1 pertinent report available currently. A retrospective review of 23 revisional tibiotalocalcaneal arthrodesis treated with rhBMP-2 (n = 7) reported that patients had a higher fusion rate than controls (n = 16; 71.4% vs 68.8%).[51] However, the time to union was longer in the rhBMP-2 group (184 vs 115.2 days).[51]

BONE MORPHOGENETIC PROTEINS IN TIBIAL NONUNIONS

Nonunions remain a challenging postoperative complication of tibial fracture repair, with 1 report indicating a failure rate of 8.9%.[52] Although bone grafting and exchange nailing constitute the standard of care, these techniques are not without difficulties. Rinjbern and van Linge reported failure to achieve union in 6% of 48 attempted revisions using central intramedullary grafting and Wiss and Stetson experienced a failure rate of 10.7% in a group of 47 revisions with a reamed intermedullary nailing technique.[52] Limited reports exist to indicate that platelet-rich plasma injections offer significant clinical advantages in the treatment of nonunions.[53,54]

BMPs have been proposed as an adjunct for the treatment of tibial nonunion. Azad and colleagues[55] studied the effect of rhBMP-2 in bony healing for a segmental femoral defect in normal and diabetic rat models. Radiographic scoring demonstrated statistically significant differences in bone healing at 3 weeks in the group without diabetes mellitus ($P<.012$) and at 6 weeks in both the diabetes and no diabetes groups ($P<.001$ and $P<.005$, respectively). On histomorphometric analysis at both 3 and 6 weeks, significant ($P<.001$) improvements in new bone formation were seen in the rhBMP-2 group, compared with the control group. Platelet endothelial cell adhesion molecule-1 staining at 3 weeks showed a 3-fold increase in the mean number of vessels for the rhBP-2 group compared with the control group (12.76 $\pm$ 5.43/mm^2 and 4.49 $\pm$ 1.89/mm^2, respectively). These results indicate the possible clinical potential of rhBMP-2 for combating nonunion complications, especially in diabetic patients, whose comorbidity confers an added obstacle to bone healing (**Fig. 1**).

Literature regarding the clinical use of BMP-2 in tibial nonunions is sparse. In a study of 118 long bone nonunion patients wherein 50 received autogenous bone grafts and 68 received autogenous bone graft plus 1.5 mg/mL rhBMP-2, Takemoto and colleagues[56] found no differences in healing or time to union. Tressler and colleagues[57] found no differences in long bone healing in a study of 19 nonunion revisions using rhBMP-2 on an absorbable collagen sponge and 74 revisions using autologous iliac crest bone graft, suggesting that BMP may be a suitable alternative to the current gold standard. In a study of 9 patients presenting with tibial nonunions

---

nonunion at 1 year postoperatively, as seen on anteroposterior (A) and lateral (B) views of the ankle. Nonunion treatment included placement of recombinant human bone morphogenetic protein-2 on an absorbable collagen sponge with plating of the fibula (C–F). Follow-up films demonstrate union of the tibia and fibula at 1 month after revision surgery, as seen on anteroposterior (G) and lateral (H) views of the ankle.

with at least 4 failed revisions each, all patients were treated with a combined radio-immunoassay (RIA) graft and intramedullary nail fixation approach with an rhBMP-2 adjunct to enhance osteoinduction. All patients achieved union between 11 and 59 weeks with the mean time to union at 27.6 weeks.[58] In a comparative study of 23 patients undergoing revision for failed fusion attempts, 7 patients underwent revision with BMP and 16 underwent revision without it.[51] For 68.8% of the non-BMP group and 71.4% of the BMP group, the result was a stable, functional limb as indicated by endpoint criteria of successful fusion and time to fusion. Time to radiographic ankle union was 115.2 and 184.0 days for the non-BMP and BMP groups, respectively. Based on limited studies of the role of BMPs in bony healing in tibiae, further investigation is warranted to determine the potential of rhBMP-2 as an adjunct to improve outcomes of recalcitrant tibial nonunion cases.[51,59]

COST

Cost effectiveness has to be considered in any procedure, but is particularly important in adjunctive treatment. There have been no studies investigating the cost effectiveness in hindfoot arthrodesis treated with rhBMP-2; however, the success of treatment with rhBMP-2 will provide huge cost savings over situations in which the bone does not heal. Alt and colleagues[60] 2009 found this concept to be valid when they reported the costs saved by treating Gustilo grade III open fractures of the tibia with rhBMP-2. Despite the high upfront direct cost of rhBMP-2, patients with faster healing times saved cost by reductions in work productivity losses.[60]

COMPLICATIONS

Complications from rhBMP-2 do exist, yet adverse events of rhBMP-2 specific to hindfoot arthrodesis remain unclear. When using rhBMP-2 in ankle and hindfoot fusion, Bibbo and colleagues[49] 2009 reported no complications that were attributable to the use of rhBMP-2. However, there was a 4% nonunion rate, a 3% wound complication rate, and a 1.5% infection rate, which were deemed acceptable given the high-risk patient population.[49] Rearick and colleagues[61] 2014 found similar adverse event rates owing to rhBMP-2 in foot and ankle fusions and fracture nonunions. In the treatment of complex tibial plateau fractures, heterotopic bone developed more frequently in patients receiving rhBMP-2.[62] Furthermore, there have been numerous complications reported in the spine literature, including ectopic epidural bone formation, bone resorption and remodeling at site of application, neurologic impairment, painful seroma, hematoma, and neck swelling.[47,63–66]

SUMMARY

Despite advances in our understanding of bone healing physiology and surgical techniques, delayed union and nonunion still occur at a considerable rate after the treatment of hindfoot arthrodesis. Although bone graft has been used frequently, there is increasing appeal of BMPs owing to the morbidity associated with harvesting bone graft and the innate osteoinductive abilities of BMPs. Effective treatment of nonunions with BMPs has been shown in multiple animal studies. Although limited in number, human clinical studies using BMPs to treat nonunions have also shown success. The only study investigating the use of rhBMP-2 in hindfoot arthrodesis found a significant increase in the fusion rate compared with controls. In addition, treatment with BMPs is cost effective and the complications from their use remain low. Overall, rhBMP-2 is a safe and effective bone-healing adjunct in hindfoot arthrodesis surgery.

ACKNOWLEDGMENTS

The authors acknowledge that considerable work was done on this article by the following individuals: Kristen Pacific, Research Fellow, Department of Orthopaedics, Rutgers New Jersey Medical School, Newark, NJ and Maximilian F. Muñoz, Research Fellow, Department of Orthopaedics, Rutgers New Jersey Medical School, Newark, NJ.

REFERENCES

1. Lopez R, Singh T, Banga S, et al. Subtalar joint arthrodesis. Clin Podiatr Med Surg 2012;29(1):67–75.
2. Saltzman CL, Fehrle MJ, Cooper RR, et al. Triple arthrodesis: twenty-five and forty-four-year average follow-up of the same patients. J Bone Joint Surg Am 1999;81(10):1391–402.
3. RFt Pell, Myerson MS, Schon LC. Clinical outcome after primary triple arthrodesis. J Bone Joint Surg Am 2000;82(1):47–57.
4. Clain MR, Baxter DE. Simultaneous calcaneocuboid and talonavicular fusion. Long-term follow-up study. J Bone Joint Surg Br 1994;76(1):133–6.
5. Easley ME, Trnka HJ, Schon LC, et al. Isolated subtalar arthrodesis. J Bone Joint Surg Am 2000;82(5):613–24.
6. Davies MB, Rosenfeld PF, Stavrou P, et al. A comprehensive review of subtalar arthrodesis. Foot Ankle Int 2007;28(3):295–7.
7. Diezi C, Favre P, Vienne P. Primary isolated subtalar arthrodesis: outcome after 2 to 5 years followup. Foot Ankle Int 2008;29(12):1195–202.
8. Herrera-Perez M, Andarcia-Banuelos C, Barg A, et al. Comparison of cannulated screws versus compression staples for subtalar arthrodesis fixation. Foot Ankle Int 2015;36(2):203–10.
9. Flemister AS Jr, Infante AF, Sanders RW, et al. Subtalar arthrodesis for complications of intra-articular calcaneal fractures. Foot Ankle Int 2000;21(5):392–9.
10. Haskell A, Pfeiff C, Mann R. Subtalar joint arthrodesis using a single lag screw. Foot Ankle Int 2004;25(11):774–7.
11. Russotti GM, Cass JR, Johnson KA. Isolated talocalcaneal arthrodesis. A technique using moldable bone graft. J Bone Joint Surg Am 1988;70(10):1472–8.
12. Crevoisier X. The isolated talonavicular arthrodesis. Foot Ankle Clin 2011;16(1):49–59.
13. Chiodo CP, Martin T, Wilson MG. A technique for isolated arthrodesis for inflammatory arthritis of the talonavicular joint. Foot Ankle Int 2000;21(4):307–10.
14. Ljung P, Kaij J, Knutson K, et al. Talonavicular arthrodesis in the rheumatoid foot. Foot Ankle 1992;13(6):313–6.
15. Chen CH, Huang PJ, Chen TB, et al. Isolated talonavicular arthrodesis for talonavicular arthritis. Foot Ankle Int 2001;22(8):633–6.
16. Toolan BC, Sangeorzan BJ, Hansen ST Jr. Complex reconstruction for the treatment of dorsolateral peritalar subluxation of the foot. Early results after distraction arthrodesis of the calcaneocuboid joint in conjunction with stabilization of, and transfer of the flexor digitorum longus tendon to, the midfoot to treat acquired pes planovalgus in adults. J Bone Joint Surg Am 1999;81(11):1545–60.
17. Frey C, Halikus NM, Vu-Rose T, et al. A review of ankle arthrodesis: predisposing factors to nonunion. Foot Ankle Int 1994;15(11):581–4.
18. Bibbo C, Anderson RB, Davis WH. Complications of midfoot and hindfoot arthrodesis. Clin Orthop Relat Res 2001;(391):45–58.
19. Chahal J, Stephen DJ, Bulmer B, et al. Factors associated with outcome after subtalar arthrodesis. J Orthop Trauma 2006;20(8):555–61.

20. Ishikawa SN, Murphy GA, Richardson EG. The effect of cigarette smoking on hindfoot fusions. Foot Ankle Int 2002;23(11):996–8.
21. Cobb TK, Gabrielsen TA, Campbell DC 2nd, et al. Cigarette smoking and nonunion after ankle arthrodesis. Foot Ankle Int 1994;15(2):64–7.
22. Myers TG, Lowery NJ, Frykberg RG, et al. Ankle and hindfoot fusions: comparison of outcomes in patients with and without diabetes. Foot Ankle Int 2012; 33(1):20–8.
23. Jaakkola JI, Mann RA. A review of rheumatoid arthritis affecting the foot and ankle. Foot Ankle Int 2004;25(12):866–74.
24. El-Amin SF, Hogan MV, Allen AA, et al. The indications and use of bone morphogenetic proteins in foot, ankle, and tibia surgery. Foot Ankle Clin 2010;15(4): 543–51.
25. Pollock R, Alcelik I, Bhatia C, et al. Donor site morbidity following iliac crest bone harvesting for cervical fusion: a comparison between minimally invasive and open techniques. Eur Spine J 2008;17(6):845–52.
26. Pinzur MS. Orthobiologics in Foot and ankle surgery. Curr Orthop Pract 2013; 24(5):457–60.
27. Urist MR. Bone: formation by autoinduction. Science 1965;150(3698):893–9.
28. Abe E. Function of BMPs and BMP antagonists in adult bone. Ann N Y Acad Sci 2006;1068:41–53.
29. Wang EA, Rosen V, D'Alessandro JS, et al. Recombinant human bone morphogenetic protein induces bone formation. Proc Natl Acad Sci U S A 1990;87(6):2220–4.
30. Kawabata M, Imamura T, Miyazono K. Signal transduction by bone morphogenetic proteins. Cytokine Growth Factor Rev 1998;9(1):49–61.
31. Nohe A, Keating E, Knaus P, et al. Signal transduction of bone morphogenetic protein receptors. Cell Signal 2004;16(3):291–9.
32. Wu X, Shi W, Cao X. Multiplicity of BMP signaling in skeletal development. Ann N Y Acad Sci 2007;1116:29–49.
33. Lou J, Tu Y, Li S, et al. Involvement of ERK in BMP-2 induced osteoblastic differentiation of mesenchymal progenitor cell line C3H10T1/2. Biochem Biophys Res Commun 2000;268(3):757–62.
34. Lai CF, Cheng SL. Signal transductions induced by bone morphogenetic protein-2 and transforming growth factor-beta in normal human osteoblastic cells. J Biol Chem 2002;277(18):15514–22.
35. Groppe J, Greenwald J, Wiater E, et al. Structural basis of BMP signaling inhibition by Noggin, a novel twelve-membered cystine knot protein. J Bone Joint Surg Am 2003;85A(Suppl 3):52–8.
36. Rosen V. BMP and BMP inhibitors in bone. Ann N Y Acad Sci 2006;1068:19–25.
37. Massague J, Seoane J, Wotton D. Smad transcription factors. Genes Dev 2005; 19(23):2783–810.
38. Cheng H, Jiang W, Phillips FM, et al. Osteogenic activity of the fourteen types of human bone morphogenetic proteins (BMPs). J Bone Joint Surg Am 2003;85A(8): 1544–52.
39. Bostrom MP, Lane JM, Berberian WS, et al. Immunolocalization and expression of bone morphogenetic proteins 2 and 4 in fracture healing. J Orthop Res 1995; 13(3):357–67.
40. Geiger M, Li RH, Friess W. Collagen sponges for bone regeneration with rhBMP-2. Adv Drug Deliv Rev 2003;55(12):1613–29.
41. Lane JM, Yasko AW, Tomin E, et al. Bone marrow and recombinant human bone morphogenetic protein-2 in osseous repair. Clin Orthop Relat Res 1999;(361): 216–27.

42. Vogelin E, Jones NF, Huang JI, et al. Healing of a critical-sized defect in the rat femur with use of a vascularized periosteal flap, a biodegradable matrix, and bone morphogenetic protein. J Bone Joint Surg Am 2005;87(6):1323–31.

43. Chen X, Kidder LS, Lew WD. Osteogenic protein-1 induced bone formation in an infected segmental defect in the rat femur. J Orthop Res 2002;20(1):142–50.

44. Yasko AW, Lane JM, Fellinger EJ, et al. The healing of segmental bone defects, induced by recombinant human bone morphogenetic protein (rhBMP-2). A radiographic, histological, and biomechanical study in rats. J Bone Joint Surg Am 1992;74(5):659–70.

45. Gerhart TN, Kirker-Head CA, Kriz MJ, et al. Healing segmental femoral defects in sheep using recombinant human bone morphogenetic protein. Clin Orthop Relat Res 1993;(293):317–26.

46. Welch RD, Jones AL, Bucholz RW, et al. Effect of recombinant human bone morphogenetic protein-2 on fracture healing in a goat tibial fracture model. J Bone Miner Res 1998;13(9):1483–90.

47. McKay WF, Peckham SM, Badura JM. A comprehensive clinical review of recombinant human bone morphogenetic protein-2 (INFUSE Bone Graft). Int Orthop 2007;31(6):729–34.

48. Ong KL, Villarraga ML, Lau E, et al. Off-label use of bone morphogenetic proteins in the United States using administrative data. Spine (Phila Pa 1976) 2010;35(19):1794–800.

49. Bibbo C, Patel DV, Haskell MD. Recombinant bone morphogenetic protein-2 (rhBMP-2) in high-risk ankle and hindfoot fusions. Foot Ankle Int 2009;30(7):597–603.

50. Fourman MS, Borst EW, Bogner E, et al. Recombinant human BMP-2 increases the incidence and rate of healing in complex ankle arthrodesis. Clin Orthop Relat Res 2014;472(2):732–9.

51. DeVries JG, Nguyen M, Berlet GC, et al. The effect of recombinant bone morphogenetic protein-2 in revision tibiotalocalcaneal arthrodesis: utilization of the Retrograde Arthrodesis Intramedullary Nail database. J Foot Ankle Surg 2012;51(4):426–32.

52. Sarmiento A, Burkhalter WE, Latta LL. Functional bracing in the treatment of delayed union and nonunion of the tibia. Int Orthop 2003;27(1):26–9.

53. Bielecki T, Gazdzik TS, Szczepanski T. Benefit of percutaneous injection of autologous platelet-leukocyte-rich gel in patients with delayed union and nonunion. Eur Surg Res 2008;40(3):289–96.

54. Kanthan SR, Kavitha G, Addi S, et al. Platelet-rich plasma (PRP) enhances bone healing in non-united critical-sized defects: a preliminary study involving rabbit models. Injury 2011;42(8):782–9.

55. Azad V, Breitbart E, Al-Zube L, et al. rhBMP-2 enhances the bone healing response in a diabetic rat segmental defect model. J Orthop Trauma 2009;23(4):267–76.

56. Takemoto R, Forman J, Taormina DP, et al. No advantage to rhBMP-2 in addition to autogenous graft for fracture nonunion. Orthopedics 2014;37(6):e525–30.

57. Tressler MA, Richards JE, Sofianos D, et al. Bone morphogenetic protein-2 compared to autologous iliac crest bone graft in the treatment of long bone nonunion. Orthopedics 2011;34(12):e877–84.

58. Desai PP, Bell AJ, Suk M. Treatment of recalcitrant, multiply operated tibial nonunions with the RIA graft and rh-BMP2 using intramedullary nails. Injury 2010;41(Suppl 2):S69–71.

59. Ollivier M, Gay AM, Cerlier A, et al. Can we achieve bone healing using the diamond concept without bone grafting for recalcitrant tibial nonunions? Injury 2015; 46(7):1383–8.

60. Alt V, Donell ST, Chhabra A, et al. A health economic analysis of the use of rhBMP-2 in Gustilo-Anderson grade III open tibial fractures for the UK, Germany, and France. Injury 2009;40(12):1269–75.

61. Rearick T, Charlton TP, Thordarson D. Effectiveness and complications associated with recombinant human bone morphogenetic protein-2 augmentation of foot and ankle fusions and fracture nonunions. Foot Ankle Int 2014;35(8):783–8.

62. Boraiah S, Paul O, Hawkes D, et al. Complications of recombinant human BMP-2 for treating complex tibial plateau fractures: a preliminary report. Clin Orthop Relat Res 2009;467(12):3257–62.

63. Wong DA, Kumar A, Jatana S, et al. Neurologic impairment from ectopic bone in the lumbar canal: a potential complication of off-label PLIF/TLIF use of bone morphogenetic protein-2 (BMP-2). Spine J 2008;8(6):1011–8.

64. Benglis D, Wang MY, Levi AD. A comprehensive review of the safety profile of bone morphogenetic protein in spine surgery. Neurosurgery 2008;62(5 Suppl 2):ONS423–31 [discussion: ONS431].

65. Joseph V, Rampersaud YR. Heterotopic bone formation with the use of rhBMP2 in posterior minimal access interbody fusion: a CT analysis. Spine (Phila Pa 1976) 2007;32(25):2885–90.

66. Poynton AR, Lane JM. Safety profile for the clinical use of bone morphogenetic proteins in the spine. Spine (Phila Pa 1976) 2002;27(16 Suppl 1):S40–8.

B2A Polypeptide in Foot and Ankle Fusion

Mark Glazebrook, MSc, PhD, Dip Sports Med, MD, FRCS(C)*, Diana S. Young, BSc, MD, FRCS(C)

KEYWORDS

- B2A • AMPLEX® • Synthetic peptide • Bone graft • Ankle fusion • Arthrodesis

KEY POINTS

- B2A is a bioactive synthetic multi-domain peptide that augments osteodifferentiation via increasing endogenous cellular bone morphogenetic protein 2 by preosteoblast receptor modulation at the local arthrodesis site.
- B2A-granule is comparable with autogenous bone graft with respect to safety and efficacy.
- Use of B2A-granule in foot and ankle fusions eliminates the risk of donor site morbidity.
- B2A-granule is yet to be tested in large-scale adequately powered randomized controlled trials.

INTRODUCTION: NATURE OF THE PROBLEM

End-stage ankle and hindfoot arthritis compromises health-related quality of life.[1–5] When nonoperative treatment fails, operative management of end-stage disease commonly involves surgical arthrodesis involving rigid internal fixation and interposition of bone graft in remaining spaces at the prepared joint surfaces.[6,7] To decrease fusion nonunion, supplemental autogenous bone graft from a donor harvest site may be used. Problems associated with autogenous bone graft include pain, donor site morbidity, variable quantity and quality of graft, and additional operating time and resources associated with harvesting the autogenous bone.[8]

Bone graft substitutes are needed for foot and ankle arthrodesis to circumvent the aforementioned problems associated with autogenous bone graft. Recently, experimental spinal fusion animal models using augmentation with B2A-coated ceramic granules formulated as PREFIX® (Ferring Pharmaceuticals, Saint-Prex, Switzerland) showed B2A-coated granules have higher fusion rates than osteoconductive granules alone. This result suggested B2A is contributing to fusion outcomes.[9,10]

The authors have nothing to disclose.
Reconstructive Foot & Ankle Surgery & Orthopaedic Sports Medicine, Queen Elizabeth II Health Sciences Center, Dalhousie University, Halifax Infirmary, Room 4867, 1796 Summer Street, Halifax, Nova Scotia B3H 3A6, Canada
* Corresponding author.
E-mail address: markglazebr@ns.sympatico.ca

1083-7515/16/© 2016 Elsevier Inc. All rights reserved.

B2A is a bioactive synthetic multi-domain peptide that augments osteogenic differentiation via increasing endogenous cellular bone morphogenetic protein 2 (BMP-2) by preosteoblast receptor modulation at the local arthrodesis site.[4] BMPs, growth factors that belong to the transforming growth factor superfamily, are upregulated naturally during bone repair.[11] The empirical formula of B2A is $C_{241}H_{418}N_{66}O_{65}S_2$, and it contains 42 amino acids and 3 lysine analogue residues of 6-aminohexanoic[8] (**Fig. 1**).

The ceramic granules associated with B2A act as an osteoconductive scaffold and method of delivery from which B2A elution occurs. Once the B2A is released, interaction with BMP receptors and the cascade leading to endogenous BMP-2 augmentation follows. This process occurs locally at the fusion site where the B2A-ceramic coated granules have been delivered intraoperatively. It takes approximately 5 weeks for absorption of B2A itself once it enters the general circulation. Over time the ceramic granule scaffold undergoes reabsorption and replacement with bridging bone.[8]

Investigations evaluating inflammatory response associated with B2A-coated ceramic granules have demonstrated no evidence of inflammatory initiation via leukocyte recruitment or endothelial cell activation. High biocompatibility of B2A and B2A-coated ceramic granules was shown.[12,13]

SURGICAL TECHNIQUE
Subtalar Arthrodesis Using B2A

The following is an overview of the surgical technique of subtalar arthrodesis incorporating B2A-granule at the fusion site.

Indications

- Failure of nonsurgical management of subtalar end-stage arthritis.

Preoperative Planning

- Weight-bearing subtalar joint radiographs, including anteroposterior, lateral, and oblique Broden views.
- Computed tomography (CT) scan of hindfoot.
- Single-photon emission CT to rule out other focus of arthritis in the midfoot and ensure area to be fused is active.

Prep and Patient Positioning

- Anesthesia: regional, spinal, or general
- Preoperative prophylactic antibiotics before incision
- Lateral decubitus positioning
- Tourniquet inflated to 350 mm Hg

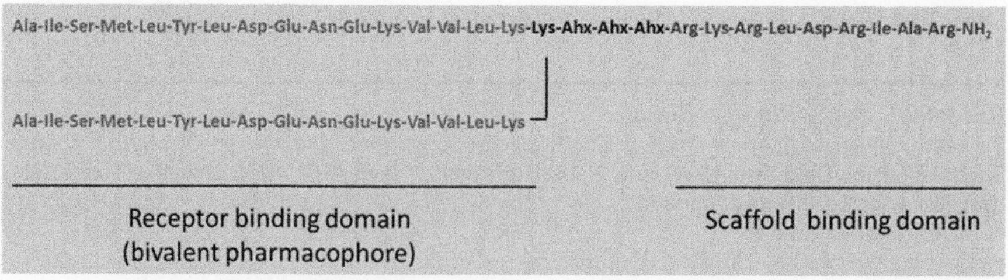

Ala-Ile-Ser-Met-Leu-Tyr-Leu-Asp-Glu-Asn-Glu-Lys-Val-Val-Leu-Lys-**Lys-Ahx-Ahx-Ahx**-Arg-Lys-Arg-Leu-Asp-Arg-Ile-Ala-Arg-NH$_2$

Ala-Ile-Ser-Met-Leu-Tyr-Leu-Asp-Glu-Asn-Glu-Lys-Val-Val-Leu-Lys ⎤

| Receptor binding domain (bivalent pharmacophore) | Scaffold binding domain |

Fig. 1. The nature of B2A. (*From* Glazebrook M, Younger A, Zamora P, et al. B2A peptide bone graft substitute: literature review, biology and use for hindfoot fusions. Curr Orthop Pract 2013;24(5):483; with permission.)

Surgical Approach and Procedure

- Lateral incision directly over sinus tarsi from tip of fibula to base of fourth metatarsal.
- Soft tissue dissection to sinus tarsi.
- Identification of subtalar joint with intraoperative image intensifier.
- Preparation of subtalar joint with osteotomes, curettes, rongeurs via decortication of remaining cartilage to subchondral bone.
- Avoid use of high-speed burrs to prevent excessive heat at fusion site, which could compromise bony union.
- Forage prepared joint surfaces with 2-mm drill bit.
- Administration of B2A.
- B2A-granule provided in preprepared kit containing one vial of lyophilized B2A peptide and porous granules (80% tricalcium phosphate/20% hydroxyapatite).
- B2A coating concentration of 225 μg/cm^3 to formulate 5.0 cm^3 of graft material.
- Fixation of joint with large fragment cannulated, partially threaded screws.
- Screws placed perpendicular to posterior facet across the fusion site entering calcaneus at heel and directed to a point just proximal to center of ankle joint medially.
- Careful irrigation so as not to wash out the B2A bone graft.
- Closure of wound with 1.0 polyglactin 910 (Vicryl) suture for deep layers, 2.0 Vicryl suture for subcutaneous layers, staples for skin.
- Sterile dressing.

Immediate Postoperative Care

- Non–weight bearing below knee cast
- Postoperative hospital stay for 1 to 3 days

Rehabilitation and Recovery

- Follow-up 10 to 14 days after surgery for cast change and suture removal.
- Non–weight bearing on operative extremity for 6 weeks.
- Progressive weight bearing at 25% body weight per week in removable cast boot.
- Wean removable cast boot after full weight bearing achieved.

COMPLICATIONS AND MANAGEMENT

Common complications and recommended management are listed in **Table 1**.

CLINICAL RESULTS IN THE LITERATURE

The promising results of animal model spinal fusion studies with B2A-coated ceramic granules have prompted investigations with B2A-coated ceramic granules in patients undergoing foot and ankle fusions. For application in the foot and ankle, B2A peptide-coated ceramic granules have been reformatted into AMPLEX® (Ferring Pharmaceuticals, Saint-Prex, Switzerland) with a coating concentration of 225 μg B2A/cm^3 ceramic granules (B2A-granule). A multicenter prospective randomized pilot clinical trial was undertaken to compare the safety and efficacy of B2A-granule with autogenous bone graft in patients undergoing foot and ankle fusions. The results were promising showing comparability in both safety and efficacy between B2A-granule and autograft in foot and ankle arthrodesis. Use of B2A-granule has the additional benefit of eliminating autogenous bone graft donor site morbidity.[14]

Patients were enrolled at 3 institutions. The study randomized 24 subjects, in a 1:1 ratio, to receive either autograft or B2A-coated ceramic granules. The average age of

Table 1	
Common complications and recommended management in foot and ankle fusion	
Complication	Management
Nonunion: diagnosis made after 6 mo by CT scan	Revision arthrodesis
Malunion	Revision arthrodesis
Intraoperative fracture	Fixation of fracture
Wound healing	Wound care
Incomplete relief of pain	Pain management; possible revision arthrodesis
Ipsilateral periarticular hindfoot arthritis	Arthrodesis after failure of nonsurgical management

Adapted from Glazebrook M, Younger A, Zamora P, et al. B2A peptide bone graft substitute: literature review, biology and use for hindfoot fusions. Curr Orthop Pract 2013;24(5):482–6; with permission.

patients receiving autogenous graft and B2A was bone graft was 54.5 years ($\pm$14.3) and 57.9 years ($\pm$14.0), respectively. In this study, the primary outcome measure was CT-defined fusion at 6 months. CT scan slices were used to quantitate the percentage fusion across the joint. At 6 months, the B2A-granule group had a higher average percent fusion (83.7 12.2% vs 75.2 22.0%). An independent, blinded radiologist interpreted all radiographic data. The radiologist was board certified and fellowship trained.

Clinical outcomes were assessed using the ankle osteoarthritis scale (AOS) questionnaire. Both the B2A-ganule group and the autograft group had improvements in the pain and disability scores over the course of the study. Pain scores were lowest at 6 weeks and improved and plateaued thereafter toward the end of the study (12 months). Patients receiving B2A did not have graft harvest-site pain. Graft harvest-site pain affected only autograft patients. In this group, graft-site pain was reported at 6 weeks (1 of 11 patients), 3 months (2 of 12 patients), and 6 months (2 of 12 patients). The maximum graft-site pain in any subject (5 on a 0–10 scale) was found in the 1 patient reporting pain at 6 weeks.

The obvious weakness of the current clinical literature on B2A as a safe and effective bone graft substitute is limited data, with only a single pilot study with insufficient sample size published. Although not statistically significant, the pilot study is supportive of a larger, statistically powered, randomized controlled trial that has currently been approved by the US Food and Drug Administration and scheduled to commence in 2017 to determine whether B2A-granule has an equivalent safety and efficacy profile compared with autograft (**Box 1**).

Box 1
Results of prospective pilot study of B2A-coated ceramic granules compared with autograft for ankle and hindfoot arthrodesis
• Similar radiographic fusion success (100% in B2A-granule group, 92% autograft)
• Improvement in pain and disability scores, both groups
• Graft harvest-site pain only in autograft-treated patients
• No adverse events in either group
Adapted from Glazebrook M, Younger A, Wing K, et al. A prospective pilot study of B2A-coated ceramic granules (Amplex) compared to autograft for ankle and hindfoot arthrodesis. Foot Ankle Int 2013;34(8):1055–63; with permission.

SUMMARY

B2A is a bioactive synthetic multi-domain peptide that augments osteodifferentiation via increasing endogenous cellular BMP-2 by preosteoblast receptor modulation at the local arthrodesis site.[4] B2A-granule is comparable with autogenous bone graft with respect to safety and efficacy. Use of B2A-granule in foot and ankle fusions eliminates the risk of donor site morbidity. B2A-granule is yet to be tested in large-scale adequately powered randomized controlled trials.

REFERENCES

1. Boone DW. Complications of iliac crest graft and bone grafting alternatives in foot and ankle surgery. Foot Ankle Clin 2003;8(1):1–14.
2. Chou LB, Mann RA, Coughlin MJ, et al. Stress fracture as a complication of autogenous bone graft harvest from the distal tibia. Foot Ankle Int 2007;28(2): 199–201.
3. DeOrio JK, Farber DC. Morbidity associated with anterior iliac crest bone grafting in foot and ankle surgery. Foot Ankle Int 2005;26(2):147–51.
4. Lin X, Guo H, Takahashi K, et al. B2A as a positive BMP receptor modulator. Growth Factors 2012;30(3):149–57.
5. Glazebrook M, Daniels T, Younger A, et al. Comparison of health-related quality of life between patients with end-stage ankle and hip arthrosis. J Bone Joint Surg Am 2008;90(3):499–505.
6. Maurer RC, Cimino WR, Cox CV, et al. Transarticular cross-screw fixation. A technique of ankle arthrodesis. Clin Orthop Relat Res 1991;(268):56–64.
7. Bednarz PA, Monroe MT, Manoli A 2nd. Triple arthrodesis in adults using rigid internal fixation: an assessment of outcome. Foot Ankle Int 1999;20(6):356–63.
8. Glazebrook M, Younger A, Zamora P, et al. B2A peptide bone graft substitute: literature review, biology and use for hindfoot fusions. Curr Orthop Pract 2013; 24(5):482–6.
9. Smucker JD, Bobst JA, Petersen EB, et al. B2A peptide on ceramic granules enhance posterolateral spinal fusion in rabbits compared with autograft. Spine 2008;33(12):1324–9.
10. Cunningham BW, Atkinson BL, Hu N, et al. Ceramic granules enhanced with B2A peptide for lumbar interbody spine fusion: an experimental study using an instrumented model in sheep: laboratory investigation. J Neurosurg Spine 2009;10(4): 300–7.
11. Chen D, Zhao M, Mundy GR. Bone morphogenetic proteins. Growth Factors 2004;22(4):233–41.
12. Liu Y, Lin X, Takahashi K, et al. B2A, a receptor modulator, increases the growth of pluripotent and preosteoblast cells through bone morphogenetic protein receptors. Growth Factors 2012;30(6):410–7.
13. Zamora PO, Lin X, Liu Y, et al. Nonclinical assessment of tumor growth enhancement potential by B2A-coated ceramic granules used in arthrodesis. Int J Toxicol 2013;32(2):146–53.
14. Glazebrook M, Younger A, Wing K, et al. A prospective pilot study of B2A-coated ceramic granules (Amplex) compared to autograft for ankle and hindfoot arthrodesis. Foot Ankle Int 2013;34(8):1055–63.

Orthobiologics in the Foot and Ankle

H. Thomas Temple, MD[a],*, Theodore I. Malinin, MD[b]

KEYWORDS

- Cartilage particulate • Micronized bone • Osteoprogenitor stem cells • Amnion

KEY POINTS

- Many allogeneic biologic materials, by themselves or in combination with cells or cell products, may be transformative in healing or regeneration of musculoskeletal bone and soft tissues.
- By reconfiguring the size, shape, and methods of tissue preparation to improve deliverability and storage, unique iterations of traditional tissue scaffolds have emerged.
- This improvement, combined with new cell technologies, has shaped an exciting platform of regenerative products that are effective and provide a bridge to newer and better methods of providing care for orthopedic foot and ankle patients.

INTRODUCTION

Biologic materials play an important and increasing role in musculoskeletal repair and regeneration in general; this is especially true in the foot and ankle. Advances in stem cell recovery, isolation, and processing combined with autogeneic, allogeneic, and synthetic scaffolds present new and exciting opportunities to address challenging clinical problems like full-thickness cartilage defects, segmental bone loss, pseudoarthroses, and delayed wound healing.

This review focuses on select cartilage, bone and soft tissue repair, and regeneration strategies. Many recent developments and commercial products, although encouraging, lack sufficient basic scientific foundation and adequate clinical outcome data. The strengths and limitations of the techniques and products are discussed, and representative commercial products are compared.

CARTILAGE

A significant number of techniques are coupled with biologic materials for full-thickness cartilage defects.[1] Successful outcomes are reported with microfracture

The authors have nothing to disclose.
[a] Orthopaedic Surgery, Nova Southeastern University, 3301 College Avenue, Fort Lauderdale, FL 33314-7796, USA; [b] Department of Orthopaedic Surgery, University of Miami Miller School of Medicine, 1951 NW 7th Ave., Miami, FL 33136, USA
* Corresponding author.
E-mail address: htemple@nova.edu

alone, but many of the defects, on reinspection, are incompletely healed,[2] and the resulting fibrocartilage lacks the biomechanical properties to satisfy the demands of joint function.[3,4] Although some, using T2 mapping to assess repair cartilage after microfracture, report good results along with improved functional scores,[5] short and intermediate magnetic resonance studies by others observe the resulting cartilage to be inferior to the adjacent normal cartilage.[6] Other biologic techniques include autogeneic cartilage transfer (mosaicplasty), allogeneic cartilage transfer (fresh and cryopreserved), and autologous chondrocyte transplantation.

Cartilage Graft

Mosaicplasty is a consideration for small and intermediate-size defects but is limited and complicated by donor site availability. The reconstruction is hardly congruent but remodels over time resulting in good short-term and intermediate-term results.

Structural cartilage allografts for intermediate and large defects involve both fresh and cryopreserved tissues. Cryopreserved grafts heal well and in the short and intermediate term produce acceptable functional results. Ultimately, however, they fail because the chondrocytes do not survive. Chondrocyte damage is thought to occur during the slow rate freezing process. The theory behind slow rate freezing with a cryopreservative is to limit the amount of heat released from the cell that ultimately results in crystallization and cell damage. Although techniques exist to reduce the rate of cell freezing down to $-150°C$ in an attempt to limit the rate of cellular heat release, they do not eliminate the phenomenon and subsequent crystallization. Most isolated cells treated in this fashion survive thawing and appear to grow normally in culture. These chondrocytes in tissue, however, do not sustain normal cell function over time, and arthrosis supervenes.[7] Other factors may contribute to cell demise, such as selection of cryopreservation alternatives, surgical technique, joint congruity, the relative health of the seemingly normal adjacent cartilage, and the underlying subchondral bone.

Alternatively, fresh grafts represent the gold standard of cartilage repair and can produce excellent long-term results in select individuals. The primary limitation of this technique is graft availability and variability in processing techniques, principally, the time interval between recovery and transplantation. Chondrocyte viability decreases significantly after 21 days in primary culture based on ex vivo and reimplantation studies.[8]

Recent investigations using particulate cartilage as a structural and potentially inductive matrix after microfracture show promising results in preclinical and early clinical studies.

Cellular Therapy for Cartilage Regeneration

Cellular therapies for cartilage regeneration are not new. Autologous cartilage cell therapy (Carticel) is a long-standing commercial product. This technique requires recovery of cells from the joint, ex vivo growth and expansion, and reintroduction into the cartilage defect. Some investigators advocate this technique for patients who do not respond to microfracture for osteochondral defects in the talus.[9] Early results were encouraging, but the fundamental lack of an associated matrix on which the cells grow in vivo may be a limitation to this strategy. Stem cell therapies with or without a matrix have not been adequately studied to comment on their efficacy.

Particulate Cartilage Allografts

In the foot and ankle, particulate cartilage allografts are attractive for small and intermediate-size osteochondral defects. These allografts can be introduced arthroscopically, produce hyalinelike cartilage matrix, appear to remodel over time, and have shown good and excellent short-term outcomes.[10] Relative to fresh and cryopreserved allografts and autologous cellular strategies, they are also relatively inexpensive.[11]

The biological basis is substantiated in several studies. The observation of a hyaline-like material forming in large full-thickness osteochondral defects in nonhuman primates set the stage for further investigation of this material.[10] In an in vitro study by Cheng and colleagues,[11] incubation of adipose stem cells with a lyophilized cartilage particle resulted in substantial upregulation of type II collagen, and the resulting cellular morphology and matrix was reminiscent of that observed in hyalinelike articular cartilage. In the same study, defects were made in the medial femoral condyles of rabbits (full-thickness cartilage defects). In comparing the control full-thickness cartilage defect with defects filled with particulate cartilage, there were striking histologic differences. In the control, there was a thin layer of predominately fibrous tissue in the defect (fibrocartilage) versus robust chondrocytes in an abundant matrix that was similar to adjacent normal hyaline cartilage in the treatment group. In addition, there was persistent upregulation of cartilage phenotypic markers, collagen IIa, and aggrecan.[12]

In anecdotal, unpublished reports, particulate cartilage was used in treating damaged cartilage in the first metatarsal phalangeal joint after cheilectomy. A clinically important site of particulate transplantation is the talus, wherein select patients with contained and small osteochondral defects treated with cartilage particles can obtain early and sustained symptomatic relief of pain and exhibit hyalinelike cartilage matrix.

In one study, smaller pore sizes used in synthetic scaffolds seemed to influence stem cell differentiation toward chondrocytes.[13] This finding may be the basis of improved chondrogenesis after microfracture and the use of micronized particles of allogeneic cartilage in nonhuman primates. Similar to experimental and clinical observations in bone, the juxtaposition of small particles seems to create a microporous structure that may influence stem cell differentiation and migration. Magnetic resonance studies, specifically proton sequences, of patient's knees after particulate cartilage repair have found inhomogeneity and slightly lower signal than normal cartilage. Also observed was decreased inflammation in the surrounding subchondral bone and remodeling of the tidemark line (T Subawong, MR imaging of BioCartilage augmented microfracture surgery utilizing 2D MOCART and KOOS scores, unpublished data, 2015).

Experimental models using cells and growth factors (transforming growth factor–β) showed substantial upregulation of proteoglycan production when compared with use of the particulate matrix alone[10] (**Table 1**).

BONE

Historically, structural and particulate bone allografts were used for closed and open segment defects. Structural autograft and allograft bone have been the mainstay for segmental defects in bone. In the foot and ankle, they serve as structural support and inductive scaffolds for bone replacement in procedures such as metatarsal phalangeal fusion after failed hemijoint implants with significant shortening, osteotomy wedges for midfoot alignment corrections, hindfoot procedures to correct alignment and height, and for segmental metatarsal defects after tumor resection and trauma.

For closed-segment defects, there are several options, both biologic and synthetic. Biologic options include both autograft and allograft bone. In the foot and ankle, autograft bone is typically recovered from the distal tibia or iliac crest depending on the size of the defect and the surgeon's preference. Autograft bone is alleged to be the gold standard of grafting material but has significant limitations, which include donor

Table 1
Overview of commercial stem cell products

Name, Distributor	Description	Processor	Cell Origin	Cell Counts	Indications	Delivery	OC/OI/OG
Via Graft and Via Form, Vivex/ UMTB Biomedical, Inc	Combination product with vial of cryopreserved viable cells, bone gel, and particulate blend packaged separately to be combined at back table	UMTB	Bone marrow of vertebral bodies	At least 150,000 cells/ mL, supra physiologic levels of OPCs and MIAMI cells	Bone void filler	Cryopreserved; bone gel jar, particulate bone jar and cell vial, DMSO free	OC, OI potential, OG
Map3, RTI	Combination product with vial of cryopreserved viable cells and bone chips packaged separately to be combined at back table	RTI Biologics	?	?	?	Cryopreserved; bone chips in plastic vial, cells in vial	OC, OI potential, OG
Trinity Evolution Orthofix	Cancellous bone matrix, demineralized cortical bone, viable MSCs and OPCs.	MTF	Bone	Guaranteed a minimum of 250,000 cells/mL, of which at least 50,000 are MSCs and/or OPCs	Allograft intended for the treatment of musculoskeletal defects	Cryopreserved; bone chips delivered in a plastic vial with DMSO	Yes
Trinity Elite, Orthofix	Third-generation moldable allograft with viable cells	MTF	Bone	Guaranteed a minimum of 500,000 cells/mL, of which at least 100,000 are MSCs and/or OPCs	Allograft intended for the treatment of musculoskeletal defects	Cryopreserved; bone chips delivered in a plastic vial with DMSO	Yes

Product	Description	Source	Tissue	Cell numbers	Intended use	Storage/delivery	
Osteocel Plus, Nuvasive	Cancellous bone matrix, demineralized cortical bone, viable MSCs and OPCs	AlloSource or LifeLink	Bone	Confirm a minimum of 250,000 cells/mL (including MSCs and OPCs) or 50,000/mL, conflicting literature	This product is restricted to homologous use for the repair, replacement or reconstruction of musculoskeletal defects	Cryopreserved; bone chips delivered in a plastic vial with DMSO	Yes
Biomet Cellentra, VCBM	Viable Cell Bone Matrix; Viable osteogenic cells, demineralized component, and a cancellous bone matrix	Tissue Bank International	Bone	250,000 cells/mL including MSCs, OPCs and preosteoblasts	Intended for homologous use in the repair, replacement, reconstruction, or supplementation of the recipient's tissue in musculoskeletal defects	Cryopreserved; bone chips delivered in a plastic vial with DMSO	Yes
Allostem, Allosource	Adipose (fat) derived MSCs seeded on partially demineralized 3-dimensional cancellous bone scaffold	AlloSource	Adipose (fat) tissue	Testing showed consistent, viable cell numbers between 66,255 cells/mL ± 27,696 from 103 donors	Allograft intended for the treatment of musculoskeletal defects	Cryopreserved; chips, cubes, dowels, or strips delivered in a pouch or vial with DMSO	Yes
ViviGen, DePuy Synthes	Cryopreserved live viable cells within a cortical cancellous bone matrix with demineralized bone, delivering all properties required for bone formation	Lifenet	Bone	?	Allograft intended for the repair or reconstruction of musculoskeletal defects	Cryopreserved; delivered in DMSO and Human serum albumin; delivered in a ported pouch	Yes

(continued on next page)

Table 1
(continued)

Name, Distributor	Description	Processor	Cell Origin	Cell Counts	Indications	Delivery	OC/OI/OG
BIO4, Stryker	BIO4 is a viable bone matrix containing endogenous bone-forming cells including MSCs, OPCs, osteoblasts, osteoinductive, and angiogenic growth factors. BIO4 possesses all 4 characteristics involved in bone repair and regeneration: osteoconductive, osteoinductive, osteogenic, and angiogenic.	Osiris Therapeutics	Bone	600,000 cells/mL (70% viability postthaw) including MSCs, OPCs, osteoblasts, and growth factors (claim angiogenesis)	?	Cryopreserved in DMSO, but claim no decanting is required?	Yes, plus angiogenesis

Abbreviations: MSC, mesenchymal stem cells; MTF, musculoskeletal tissue foundation; OC, osteoconductive; OI, osteoinductive; OG, osteogenic; OPC, osteoprogenitor cells; ?, not reported.

site morbidity and graft availability. Furthermore, allogenic bone particles in specific size dimensions are found to incorporate as well, and in some cases, better than autograft.[14] Knowing this, the use of autograft bone in general, and in the foot and ankle in particular, is rarely necessary.

Processing and Preparation

Scaffolds differ in many ways: processing, mineralized and demineralized, cryopreserved and freeze dried, secondary sterilization or aseptic processing, and size. Although there are inductive advantages in having small particle sizes, there is no general agreement on optimal scaffold preparation and function.

Allograft bone is available in many different preparations but in general includes fresh frozen, cryopreserved, and freeze-dried compositions; however, there are few instances or indications in which fresh frozen or cryopreserved bone is needed or used clinically. In fact, the presence of hematomyelopoietic cells in both frozen and cryopreserved bone may be detrimental to bone healing because of the possibility of evoking a host immune response in addition to the increased possibility of disease transmission. For this reason, in most, if not all circumstances, freeze-dried bone preparations are preferred. Freeze-dried bone can be either cortical, cancellous, or corticocancellous and may be structural or nonstructural. Among the nonstructural types, there is great variability regarding size and the presence or absence of demineralization. Bone demineralization is thought to mobilize bone morphogenic protein and thus create a substrate that has greater inductive osteogenic potential than nondemineralized bone. It is important to remember, however, that in the process of acid denaturation of bone, other antigens may be exposed, thus, potentially increasing immunogenicity to the substrate. Demineralization may involve the surface of bone only (partial) or the entire bone (typically <5% calcium by most standards).

Effect of Particle Size

Particle size is an important factor in the rate and quality of bone incorporation. In one study of nonhuman primates, closed-segment defects were made in the distal femoral condyles, and various sized particles were used to fill the defects, which were then compared with a control animal in which no graft material was used. Animals were killed at 6 weeks, and radiographs and histologic preparations were made and stained with hematoxylin and eosin. This study found that particle sizes between 100 and 300 μm resulted in optimal osseous incorporation compared with smaller and larger particle sizes.[15] This study was followed by another prospective nonrandomized clinical trial in human subjects with similar defects, mostly in metaphyseal region bones throughout the appendicular skeleton. Again, rapid healing was observed, usually within 6 weeks and, as anticipated, progressed from the periphery at the host bone allograft interface to the center of the graft. Also important was the observation that these bone particles did not form heterotopic bone in the soft tissues. The rate of healing and quality of the resulting bone were equal to or, in some instances, better than those cases in which autogenous bone was used.[15] These observations supported those of the preclinical study,[16] suggesting that microparticle bone in the 100- to 300-μm range by itself is a powerful inductive scaffold for bone formation. Other investigators found that particle size is an important factor in osteogenic activity of freeze-dried allogeneic bone.[17,18]

Cellular Component of Allograft

Significant variation in the types of scaffolds and composition of cells exists among the several iterations of commercial stem cell products (see **Table 1**). All cell products cited herein fall under the auspices of Tissue Rule 21 CFR 1271 and are considered "361 Human Cell and Tissue Products" meaning that they comply with 2 important conditions in addition to safety; these are minimal manipulation and homology. This definition means that the cell products are not substantially changed from their normal or natural constitution and that the cells are derived from a site (ie, bone or bone marrow) and are used in or applied to that specific site clinically.

Cell claims are different from one product to another. In some preparations, the numbers and types of cells are well understood, whereas in others, this is not the case. Moreover, it is unclear what number and types of cells alone or in combination are necessary for optimal bone healing. It is not even certain how many cells survive freezing and thawing, as most cell products rely on dimethyl sulfoxide (DMSO), which is toxic to cells and requires significant dilution before use to avoid toxicity to the recipient. Therefore, the end concentration of cells delivered to tissue for the purpose of repair is substantially less than the product specifications. For these reasons, it is difficult for the end user to have a perspective on the best product for a given patient or indication of use.

In the foot and ankle, cell matrix products may have a beneficial effect in achieving fusion in joints that are sometimes difficult to fuse, such as tibiotalar arthrodesis, talonavicular arthrodesis, or failed first metatarsophalangeal fusion with concomitant bone loss and scarred devascularized soft tissue. This finding may be especially true for stem cells that are relatively primitive insofar as they may have the capacity to repair other tissues in addition to bone such as blood vessels and nerves. Other indications for using allogeneic cell matrix products are segmental bone loss after trauma as an augment to structural grafting and for patients with significant comorbidities that adversely affect fusion, such as, rheumatoid arthritis, diabetes, vascular disease, and poorly vascularized surrounding soft tissue. The fundamental problem is precise characterization of the cells thought to be participating in the repair and the lack of clinical trials that directly compare control subjects with subjects with scaffold only and others with both scaffold and matrix. Furthermore, altering a cell in such a way that genes or microRNAs are inserted by transduction or transfection to promote osseous bone formation falls well beyond minimal manipulation as does cell expansion.

Other Scaffold

Several other scaffolds are reported that include, but are not limited to, bioglasses and ceramics. By themselves, they are not inductive but osteoconductive only. These scaffolds can also be used in combination with allogeneic bone particles or molecules, such as bone morphogenic protein in which case they also become inductive. Other potential strategies exist that combine pedestrian allograft compositions with growth factors that, in some studies, show improved bone healing. One such example is a product that combines recombinant platelet-derived growth factor with β tricalcium phosphate. In a prospective study comparing 20 patients with autologous bone graft with augment for patients undergoing foot and ankle fusion, the investigators noted equivalency between the 2 groups regarding rate of radiographic union, time to full weight bearing, and outcomes scores.[19] The use of a single molecule in supraphysiologic doses to effectively heal bone as efficiently as autologous bone graft is interesting, as bone healing involves many different molecules that appear temporally throughout the healing process.

WOUND HEALING

Many products, both biologic and nonbiologic, are used for wound healing, mostly for chronic wounds of the foot and ankle associated with diabetes, vascular insufficiency, or trauma. Discussion of all of available products, even product categories, is beyond the scope of this article. Instead, the focus is on an old remedy, placental membranes,[20,21] recently retooled and packaged in a heat stable form to treat both acute and chronic wounds, prevent adhesions, reduce inflammation, and decrease pain. These membranes are considered barriers and contain growth and anti-inflammatory factors, are immune privileged, may have antimicrobial properties, and produce local analgesic effects.[22] These membranes are not substitutes for the basic tenants of wound management, specifically, debridement, relief of pressure, restoring adequate vascular flow, and appropriate antibiotic intervention, but may play a role in improving the rate and quality of soft-tissue healing. They are powerful adjuncts to wound healing[23] (**Fig. 1**).

Placental Membrane

Placental membranes may include the chorion in addition to the amnion or the umbilical cord itself. The configuration of tissue (double folded amnion), addition of the chorion layer, or use of the umbilical cord can create tissues of greater thickness, which improve their handling characteristics and provide a mechanical contribution to a repair such as an Achilles tendon or rotator cuff. The increased tissue thickness

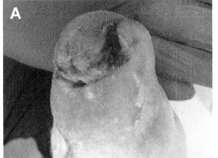
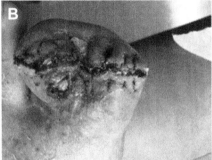
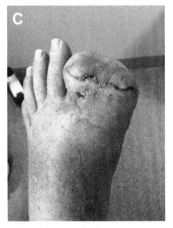

Fig. 1. (*A*) 42-year-old man with a history of a hamartoma of the great toe who underwent an amputation through the proximal interphalangeal joint that was complicated by a wound infection and osteomyelitis. (*B*) The patient underwent a revision of the distal residual digit that resulted in a wound dehiscence. (*C*) Appearance of the wound after 3 weeks of amnion therapy.

and improved handling characteristics allow for arthroscopic or laparoscopic introduction, placement, and anchoring of the tissue.

Amnion Membrane

Several companies distribute amnion tissues, most of which are freeze dried and stable at room temperature. The types of tissues and claims made by the respective companies are listed in **Table 2**.

In general, amniotic membranes are thin and contain an epithelial layer and base-
ment membrane. These membranes are generally applied to the surface of the wound,
on top of a tendon or nerve, or potentially interposed between joint surfaces. Thin
membranes are applied dry, whereas the thicker membranes may be applied and
manipulated in a wet form. In certain regions (ie, over the anterior distal leg and ankle
where wound healing complications are not infrequent after trauma and surgical procedures or over the taloachilles tendon) the application of amnion in the subcutaneous
tissue, over the tendon, and on the skin as a "biological bandage" may substantially
improve wound healing. Although, to the authors' knowledge, there are no specific reports of the use of amnion after nerve sheath tumor excision the authors' observation
is that amnion decreases postoperative pain, diminishes the intensity of neuritic pain,
and seems to restore normal function more rapidly. To validate these preliminary observations, further controlled studies are needed. Similarly, the direct application of
amnion to the posterior tibial nerve following decompression after tarsal tunnel release
acts as a barrier to scar formation and may mitigate the use of veins, for example, as a
protective barrier to scar formation and nerve dysfunction. Freeze-dried amniotic tissues have been used clinically to augment sites of nerve repair,[24] and Meng and colleagues[25] observed significant benefit in using amnion as a wrap in repairing sciatic
nerve injuries in rats. The membrane adheres intimately to the nerve and does not
require anchor sutures. The thicker membranes (double folded) or those containing
both amnion and chorion layers can be used at the site of tendon repairs to reinforce
the repair and augment wound healing. Amnion is an excellent soft tissue adjunct to
wound healing for tumors in the foot, especially in select patients who undergo resection of plantar fibromatosis in which wound healing is challenging. Finally, after radio-
therapy in the foot for malignant tumors, the authors observed improved healing and
diminished radiation fibrosis when using amnion in the operative bed and as a
bandage on the skin.

Amniotic Fluid

Amniotic fluid is also a rich source of growth and anti-inflammatory factors. Like the
placental membranes and umbilical cords, amniotic fluid is recovered from normal
38-week pregnancies before cesarean sections. Typically, 200 to 300 mL of fluid is
recovered and processed by a variety of techniques. Then, depending on whether
viable cells are claimed to be part of the product, a cryopreservative may be added,
typically DMSO. It is then stored in a frozen form and thawed immediately before use.

In our own laboratory, we identified a substantial amount of cell debris but have
been unable to isolate anything reminiscent of amniotic stem cells and conclude
that the presence of these cells in 38-week gestational amniotic fluid is rare, and
claims otherwise should be carefully scrutinized.

The amniotic fluid is generally delivered as an injection into a tendon sheath, plantar
fascia, around an inflamed nerve, or into a degenerative of inflamed joint. Zelen and
colleagues,[25] in a prospective randomized trial, used micronized amnion in fluid sus-
pension compared with lidocaine and saline and observed significant improvement in
patients receiving the amnion composition compared with controls. Werber

Table 2
Types of amnion tissues

Company	Name(s)	Sizes	Storage	Storage Timeframe
AmnioGenix	AmnioDryFlex	1.5 × 2 cm, 2 × 3 cm, 2 × 6 cm	Room temp	2 y
	AmnioExCel	15 × 20 mm, 20 × 30 mm		
Applied Biologics	XWRAP Hydro Plus	2 × 2 cm, 2 × 6 cm, 4 × 4 cm, 4 × 6 cm, 4 × 8 cm	Room temp	1 y
	XWRAP Dry			
	XWRAP ECM			
BioDlogics	Fence	2 × 3 cm, 2 × 6 cm, 4 × 4 cm, 4 × 8 cm, 10 × 10 cm	Room temp (in saline)	2 y
	DryFlex	1.5 × 2 cm, 2 × 3 cm, 2 × 6 cm, 4 × 4 cm, 4 × 8 cm	Room temp	5 y
	Optix	1.5 × 2 cm, 2 × 3 cm − 9-, 12-, and 15-mm discs		
BioTissue	Prokera	Small sizes for ophthalmic applications	−80°C	2 y
	AmnioGraft			
	AmnioGuard			
Bone Bank AlloGrafts	SteriShield II single-layer patch	1 × 1 cm, 2 × 2 cm, 4 × 4 cm, 4 × 6 cm	Room temp	3 y
	SteriShield II double-layer patch	1 × 1 cm, 2 × 2 cm, 2 × 3 cm, 4 × 4 cm, 4 × 6 cm, 4 × 8 cm		
	SteriShield II double-layer disc	10- and 16-mm discs		
Derma Sciences	Amnioexcel	1.5 × 1.5 cm, 2 × 3 cm, 4 × 4 cm, 4 × 8 cm	Room temp	2 y
MiMedx	AmnioFix Sheet	2 × 3 cm, 3 × 3 cm, 4 × 4 cm, 4 × 6 cm, 16-mm disc	Room temp	5 y
	AmnioFix Wrap	2 × 2 cm, 2 × 4 cm 4 × 6 cm		
	EpiFix	2 × 3 cm, 4 × 4 cm, 4 × 6 cm, 14-and 16-mm disc		
NuTech	NuShield	2 × 3 cm, 4 × 4 cm, 4 × 6 cm, 6 × 6 cm	Room temp	—
Regenerative Processing Plant	Cryo-Activ	2 × 2 cm, 4 × 4 cm, 4 × 6 cm, 8 × 8 cm	−80°C	1 y

(continued on next page)

Table 2
(continued)

Company	Name(s)	Sizes	Storage	Storage Timeframe
Single Source Surgical	AlloShield AlloShield Dry	1 × 1 cm, 1 × 2 cm, 2 × 2 cm, 2 × 3 cm, 2 × 4 cm, 2 × 6 cm, 4 × 4 cm, 4 × 6 cm, 4 × 8 cm, 8 × 8 cm	Rocm temp	2 y
Skye Biologics	ActiveBarrier 45 ActiveBarrier 200 OculoMatrix VisiDisc	2 × 2 cm, 2 × 4 cm, 4 × 4 cm, 4 × 6 cm, 4 × 8 cm 1 × 1 cm, 2 × 2 cm, 2 × 4 cm, 4 × 4 cm 10 mm disc	Rocm temp	5 y
Vivex	Cygnus Solo Cygnus Matrix Cygnus Max	1 × 1 cm, 1 × 2 cm, 2 × 2 cm, 2 × 3 cm, 3 × 3 cm, 3 × 4 cm, 3 × 6 cm, 3 × 8 cm, 4 × 4 cm, 4 × 6 cm, 4 × 8 cm, 7 × 7 cm, 10 × 10 cm, 10 × 12 cm, 2 × 12 cm	Rocm temp	5 y
AmnioGenix	AmnioDryFlex AmnioExCel	1.5 × 2 cm, 2 × 3 cm, 2 × 6 cm 15 × 20 mm, 20 × 30 mm	Rocm temp	2 y
Applied Biologics	XWRAP Hydro Plus XWRAP Dry XWRAP ECM	2 × 2 cm, 2 × 6 cm, 4 × 4 cm, 4 × 6 cm, 4 × 8 cm	Rocm temp	1 y
BioDlogics	Fence DryFlex Optix	2 × 3 cm, 2 × 6 cm, 4 × 4 cm, 4 × 8 cm, 10 × 10 cm 1.5 × 2 cm, 2 × 3 cm, 2 × 6 cm, 4 × 4 cm, 4 × 8 cm 1.5 × 2 cm, 2 × 3 cm – 9-, 12-, and 15-mm discs	Rocm Temp (in saline) Rocm temp	2 y 5 y
BioTissue	Prokera AmnioGraft AmnioGuard	Small sizes for ophthalmic applications	–80°C	2 y

Table 3
Various amniotic fluid products

Company	Name(s)	Description	Dilute	Storage	Sizes	Processed by	Product Positioning
Amnio-Technology	PalinGen Flow	Liquid	Yes	Frozen	S, M, L, XL	Pinnacle Transplant Technologies	Revolutionizing the way we repair nerve, tendon, ligament and soft-tissue defects. Heal faster, live better.
Amniox	Clarix FLO, Neox FLO	Particulate AM and UC	Yes	Room temp	25, 50, 100, 150 mg	TissueTech	Provide higher volumes of the critical matrix proteins innate to the tissue
BioD	BioDRestore	Morselized flowable	Yes	Frozen	S, M, L	BioDlogics	Get back in action naturally
							A better approach to regenerative medicine
	BioDFactor	Liquid	No	Frozen	S, M, L, XL		
MiMedx	EpiFix Particulate	Particulate	Yes	Room temp	40, 100, 160 mg	MiMedx Tissue Services	Dehydrated amnion/chorion
	OrthoFlo	Liquid	No	Frozen	.25, .5, 1, 2 mL		Better healing, better repair
NuTech	NuCel, ReNu	Liquid		Frozen	S, M, L, XL	WuXi AppTec	Provides an enhanced environment for tissue growth, repair, and healing
Skye	ActiveMatrix, WoundEx, PX50, ScarEx Flow	Liquid	No	Room temp	M, L, XL	Human Regenerative Technologies	The right formulation for the right indication
	CryoMatrix and RX Flow	Liquid	Yes	Frozen	M, L, XL		
	Integra BioFix Flow	Liquid	No	Room temp	M, L, XL		
Applied Biologics	FloGraft, FloGraft Freedon (Sports)	Liquid	No	Frozen	M, L, XL		Discover the power of biological healing
Vivex	AlloGen, AlloGen-LI	Liquid	No	Frozen	S, M, L, XL	UMTB	All-natural liquid matrix

demonstrated dramatic and sustained pain reduction on injecting liquid amnion into the Achilles tendon and plantar fascia in symptomatic patients.[26] Finally, Hanselman[27] in another prospective randomized study comparing steroid injections to amniotic fluid found safety and comparable efficacy.[28] Amniotic fluid can also be aerosolized and sprayed into or onto tendons or nerves alone or to augment the membranes during an open procedure. The various products are listed in **Table 3**.

SUMMARY

Many allogeneic biologic materials, by themselves or in combination with cells or cell products, may be transformative in healing or regeneration of musculoskeletal bone and soft tissues. By reconfiguring the size, shape, and methods of tissue preparation to improve deliverability and storage, unique iterations of traditional tissue scaffolds have emerged. These new iterations, combined with new cell technologies, have shaped an exciting platform of regenerative products that are effective and provide a bridge to newer and better methods of providing care for orthopedic foot and ankle patients.

REFERENCES

1. Murawski CD, Kennedy JG. Operative treatment of osteochondral lesions of the talus. J Bone Joint Surg Am 2013;95(11):1045–54.
2. Lee KB, Bai LB, Yoon TR, et al. Second-look arthroscopic findings and clinical outcomes after microfracture for osteochondral lesions of the talus. Am J Sports Med 2009;37(Suppl 1):63S–70S.
3. Carey JL. Fibrocartilage following microfracture is not as robust as native articular cartilage: commentary on an article by Aaron J. Krych, MD, et al.: "Activity levels are higher after osteochondral autograft transfer mosaicplasty than after microfracture for articular cartilage defects of the knee. A retrospective comparative study". J Bone Joint Surg Am 2012;94(11):e80.
4. Longo UG, Petrillo S, Franceschetti E, et al. Stem cells and gene therapy for cartilage repair. Stem Cells Int 2012;2012:168385.
5. Becher C, Zühlke D, Plaas C, et al. T2-mapping at 3 T after microfracture in the treatment of osteochondral defects of the talus at an average follow-up of 8 years. Knee Surg Sports Traumatol Arthrosc 2015;23(8):2406–12.
6. Ross KA, Hannon CP, Deyer TW, et al. Functional and MRI outcomes after arthroscopic microfracture for treatment of osteochondral lesions of the distal tibial plafond. J Bone Joint Surg Am 2014;96(20):1708–15.
7. Malinin TI, Mnaymneh W, Lo HK, et al. Cryopreservation of articular cartilage. Ultrastructural observations and long-term results of experimental distal femoral transplantation. Clin Orthop Relat Res 1994;303:18–32.
8. Malinin TI, Temple HT, Buck BE. Transplantation of osteochondral allografts after cold storage. J Bone Joint Surg Am 2006;88:762–70.
9. Giza E, Sullivan M, Ocel D, et al. Matrix-induced autologous chondrocyte implantation of talus articular defects. Foot Ankle Int 2010;31(9):747–53.
10. Delcroix GJ-R, D'Ippolito G, Reiner T, et al. TGF-β-3 pharmacologically active microcarriers combined with human cartilage microparticles drive MIAMI cells to a hyaline cartilage phenotype. CellR4 2015;3:e1394.
11. Hirahara AM, Mueller KW Jr. BioCartilage: a new biomaterial to treat chondral lesions. Sports Med Arthrosc 2015;23(3):143–8.

12. Cheng N, Estes BT, Awad HA, et al. Chondrogenic differentiation of adipose-derived adult stem cells by a porous scaffold derived from native articular cartilage extracellular matrix. Tissue Eng Part A 2009;15(2):231–41.
13. Di Luca A, Szlazak K, Lorenzo-Moldero I, et al. Influencing chondrogenic differentiation of human mesenchymal stromal cells in scaffolds displaying a structural gradient in pore size. Acta Biomater 2016;36:210–9.
14. Malinin TI, Carpenter EM, Temple HT. Particulate bone graft in incorporation in regeneration of osseous defects: importance of particle sizes. Open Orthop J 2007;1:19–24.
15. Temple HT, Malinin TI. Microparticulate cortical allograft: an alternative to autograft in the treatment of osseous defects. Open Orthop J 2008;2:91–6.
16. Malinin TI, Temple HT. Transplantation of allogeneic cartilage in musculoskeletal tissue. In: Malinin TI, Temple HT, editors. Musculoskeletal tissue transplantation and tissue banking. New Dehli (India): Jaypee Brothers Med. Publishers; 2013. p. 143.
17. Shapoff CA, Bowers GM, Levy B, et al. The effect of particle size on the osteogenic activity of composite grafts of allogeneic freeze-dried bone and autogenous marrow. J Periodontol 1980;51:625–30.
18. Romagnoli C, Brandi ML. Adipose mesenchymal stem cells in the field of bone tissue engineering. World J Stem Cells 2014;6:144–52.
19. Digiovanni CW, Baumhauer J, Lin SS, et al. Prospective, randomized, multi-center feasibility trial of rhPDGF-BB versus autologous bone graft in a foot and ankle fusion model. Foot Ankle Int 2011;32(4):344–54.
20. Davis JW. Skin transplantation with a review of 550 cases at the Johns Hopkins Hospital. Johns Hopkins Med J 1910;15:307–96.
21. Sabella N. Use of fetal membranes in skin grafting. Med Rec NY 1913;83:478–80.
22. Fetterolf DE, Snyder RJ. Scientific and clinical support for the use of dehydrated amniotic membrane in wound management. Wounds 2014;24:299–307.
23. Sheikh ES, Sheikh ES, Fetterolf DE. Use of dehydrated human amniotic membrane allografts to promote healing in patients with refractory non healing wounds. Int Wound J 2014;11:711–7.
24. Fairbairn NG, Ng-Glazier J, Meppelink AM, et al. Improving outcomes in immediate and delayed nerve grafting of peripheral nerve gaps using light-activated sealing of neurorrhaphy sites with human amnion wraps. Plast Reconstr Surg 2016;137:887–95.
25. Meng H, Li M, You F, et al. Assessment of processed human amniotic membrane as a protective barrier in rat model of sciatic nerve injury. Neurosci Lett 2011;496:48–53.
26. Zelen CM, Gould L, Serena TE, et al. A prospective, randomised, controlled, multi-centre comparative effectiveness study of healing using dehydrated human amnion/chorion membrane allograft, bioengineered skin substitute or standard of care for treatment of chronic lower extremity diabetic ulcers. Int Wound J 2015; 12(6):724–32.
27. Hanselman AE, Tidwell JE, Santrock RD. Cryopreserved human amniotic membrane injection for plantar fasciitis: a randomized, controlled, double-blind pilot study. Foot Ankle Int 2015;36:151–8.
28. Werber B. Amniotic tissues for the treatment of chronic plantar fasciosis and achilles tendinosis. J Sports Med (Hindawi Publ Corp) 2015;2015:219896.

Autologous Bone Graft in Foot and Ankle Surgery

Christopher P. Miller, MD[a], Christopher P. Chiodo, MD[b],*

KEYWORDS

- Autologous bone graft • Iliac crest • Proximal tibia • Calcaneus
- Reamer-Irrigator-Aspirator (RIA) • Bone healing

KEY POINTS

- Autologous graft is the gold standard choice for bone graft and may be harvested safely and quickly with the proper tools and techniques.
- Autologous graft is the only graft option that is osteogenic, osteoinductive, and osteoconductive.
- The quantity of bone graft required and the patient positioning for the primary surgery dictates the harvest site and technique.
- The graft may be harvested from several sites including the iliac crest, proximal tibia, and calcaneus and from within the intramedullary canal using a reaming device.
- Autograft is associated with donor site pain and morbidity; however, this complication is usually limited in foot and ankle surgery, as the primary surgeries rarely require large quantities of bone graft.

INTRODUCTION

Bone graft is a common adjunct procedure in orthopedic surgery used for fusions, fracture repair, and the reconstruction of skeletal defects in the foot and ankle. Autologous graft, or autograft, involves the transport of bone from a donor site to another location in the same patient. It is considered by many to be the gold standard of bone grafting, as it is provides all biologic factors required for functional graft. Further, autograft is 100% histocompatible with no risk of disease transmission.[1-7]

Autograft bone is osteogenic, providing osteoblasts and osteocytes and precursors that will form bone. Autograft bone is also osteoinductive, bringing growth factors and matrix proteins as well as signaling molecules that will facilitate bone growth. Finally, it

---

The authors have nothing to disclose.
[a] Carl J. Shapiro Department of Orthopaedics, Beth Israel Deaconess Medical Center, Boston, MA, USA; [b] Department of Orthopedic Surgery, Brigham and Women's Hospital, Boston, MA, USA
* Corresponding author.
E-mail address: cchiodo@partners.org

is osteoconductive, providing a mineral and collagen scaffold for native cells and bone healing to occur in an ordered predictable fashion.

Historically, the common autograft harvest site was the iliac crest. Early complication rates were reported to be as high as 20% to 39% for minor and 2.5% to 10% for major complications.[8–11] Combined with the lack of anatomic proximity, concerns about complications led foot and ankle surgeons to search for alternative harvest sites. These alternative sites included the proximal and distal tibia, the calcaneus, and the intramedullary canal of the tibia and femur.

Commercially available bone graft substitutes have also been developed. Although these substitutes eliminate the risk and potential morbidity associated with graft harvest, no such product is proven to be superior to autologous graft. Additionally, one other concern lies in the significant expenses when using synthetic graft options.

GRAFT COMPOSITION AND QUALITY

Cancellous autograft is the most commonly used autograft in foot and ankle surgery. This type of autograft has a high surface area and contains osteogenic cells. The lattice of trabecular bone provides access for revascularization from the native bone and rapid incorporation of the graft.[6] Cancellous graft lacks structural stability and is, therefore, not appropriate when used in isolation to sustain compressive loads. However, this lack of structure also makes it an ideal choice when filling small defects. Because of the osteogenic properties and porosity of the cancellous bone, cancellous autograft is also highly angiogenic and readily revascularized into the host bone.[6]

In contrast to cancellous bone graft, pure cortical graft offers excellent initial stability. However, this comes at the cost of slower revascularization and incorporation into the host bone because of the minimal osteogenic potential in the cortex. These types of grafts are less frequently used in the foot and ankle, usually as a composite graft to achieve early stability and with the expectation that bone healing and union may initially occur elsewhere at first. An example would be an ankle fusion that required a cortical bone graft strut for bone loss caused by asymmetric ankle arthritis.

Cortico-cancellous graft allows for a compromise between structurally weak but osteogenic cancellous graft and stable but biologically inaccessible cortical graft. These grafts are most commonly harvested from the iliac crest and may have up to 3 cortices intact depending on surgical technique.

Vascularized bone graft is much less commonly used in foot and ankle procedures. A vascularized graft is most often considered when there is concern about the quality of the native bone blood supply, as with osteonecrosis or the case of a chronic, atrophic nonunion. Because of the special nature of these grafts, they require the expertise of a microvascular-trained surgeon. In the appropriate patient, they can bring needed structure, biology, and blood flow to a biologically compromised region.[12,13]

One critical consideration lies in the graft quality. Donor sites are not equal with regard to osteogenic cellularity. In the senior author's histologic study comparing samples of bone graft harvested from the iliac crest and proximal tibia, only the iliac crest grafts contained active hematopoietic marrow (**Fig. 1**).[14] In contrast, the tibial grafts contained quiescent fat and little hematopoietic marrow. Similarly, Hyer and colleagues[15] found that marrow aspirate collected from the iliac crest had a higher concentration of mesenchymal stem osteoprogenitor cells than aspirates from the distal tibia or the calcaneus.

These findings have implications regarding bone graft and its cellular contributions to healing. Clinically, these findings support the use of hematopoietic iliac crest graft or aspirate, at least in patients at high risk for nonunion. Meanwhile, the finding that tibial

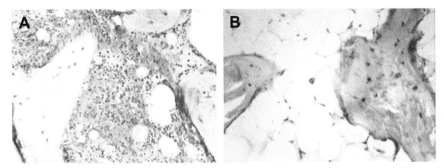

Fig. 1. Histologic slides of iliac (*A*) and tibial (*B*) bone graft. The iliac crest bone graft shows abundant osteoblasts and hematopoietic marrow. The tibial bone graft shows fatty marrow without hematopoiesis. (*From* Chiodo CP, Hahne J, Wilson MG, et al. Histological differences in iliac and tibial bone graft. Foot Ankle Int 2010;31:420; with permission.)

graft is largely devoid of hematopoiesis may support the view that autograft is not always necessary in foot and ankle reconstructions. More specifically, autograft may be replaced by allograft cancellous bone, whose osteoconductive properties may be sufficient for bony union.

AVAILABLE HARVEST SITES
Anterior Iliac Crest

The anterior iliac crest contains a large volume of cancellous bone. Dawson and colleagues[4] reported that an average of 20.7 cm³ of graft could be harvested from this region. Meanwhile, Ahlmann and colleagues[1] noted that up to 54.5 cm³ of graft could be harvested when needed to fill large bone defects after trauma.

Additionally, the iliac crest is a reliable source of cortico-cancellous structural graft.[2,3,5,7,16] The outer and inner tables of the ilium are composed of dense cortical bone with interposed cancellous bone. This composition offers structural rigidity that may be beneficial when reconstructing large defects. In the foot and ankle, this is particularly pertinent in certain fusions with bone loss. Tricortical autograft provides rich cancellous bone to facilitate fusion combined with dense cortical bone for structure. Culpan and colleagues[3] successfully revised failed total ankle replacements to fusion while preserving leg length with the use of a tricortical iliac crest. In this series, 15 of the 16 patients had successful fusion. Bhosale and colleagues[2] described the use of a tricortical graft for complex first metatarsal-phalangeal fusions after bone loss caused by removal of a prosthesis or prior Keller procedure. Nine of the 10 patients in this series progressed to fusion while restoring medial column length.

Proximal and Distal Tibial Metaphysic

The proximal and distal tibial metaphyses also contain substantial volumes of cancellous bone. Although they do not offer structural graft, the subcutaneous nature of these sites greatly facilitates harvest. Further, both sites can be readily prepared into the surgical field when performing foot and ankle procedures.

Herford and colleagues[17] reported that an average of 25 cm³ of cancellous bone could be harvested from the proximal tibia. Meanwhile, in the study by van Damme and Merkx,[18] approximately 40 cm³ was harvested without complications in a small series of 9 patients using a trephine to obtain dowels of bone from the proximal tibia. Raikin and Brislin[19] reported on harvest from the distal tibia using a 9-mm trephine and noted that 5 to 10 cm^3 of bone was routinely taken, with up to 15 cm^3 if needed, in a series of 68 hindfoot fusions and 2 revision midfoot fusions. Similarly, O'Keeffe and colleagues[20] reported sufficient harvest quantity from the proximal tibia, with very low (1.3%) donor site morbidity.

Calcaneus

The posterior calcaneal tuberosity lies in closest proximity to the foot when compared with other harvest sites. As such, it is particularly useful for midfoot and forefoot fusions and fracture repair. Biddinger and colleagues[21] reported a technique in which up to three 8-mm trephine cores were harvested from the calcaneus with minimal morbidity. Both the medial and lateral cortices of the tuberosity were perforated in this study. Meanwhile, Roukis[22] used a similar technique without penetrating the medial cortex to obtain the graft. Finally, DiDomenico and Haro[23] reported harvesting 3 to 5 cm^3 using a corticotomy and curettage technique with only 2 to 3 minutes of extra surgical time.

Long-Bone Medullary Harvest

The use of a reamer-irrigator-aspirator (RIA; DePuy Synthes, New Brunswick, NJ) was originally designed to decrease the risk of thromboembolic complications with traditional reaming for femoral and tibial nails. It was theorized that aspirating while reaming would decrease the risk of fat emboli syndrome. A benefit of the procedure was the ability to save the reamed material and collect large quantities of bone graft. Harvest volumes of up to 30 to 90 cm^3 have been reported from the femur.[4,7,24] Molecular and cell biology studies found similar quantities of osteogenic cells and factors in the graft obtained using the RIA technique when compared with the iliac crest.[4,25,26]

INDICATIONS/CONTRAINDICATIONS

When it comes to the use of autograft, the surgeon must answer several questions. First, is autograft even necessary? In a healthy individual undergoing fusion or fracture repair in which there are minimal bony defects or voids, autograft may not be needed. In the authors' experience, most fusions have regions of incongruity; therefore, some type of graft is usually indicated. Given the low complication rates associated with modern harvests and the poor muscular envelope around the foot and ankle, the authors do routinely use autograft.

The second question the surgeon must answer is how much graft is needed? For small defects such as those encountered in midfoot and forefoot fusions, the volume harvested from the calcaneus or tibia should suffice. For larger defects such as those associated with complex hindfoot and ankle fusions, iliac crest or RIA should be considered.

The third question is whether or not structural graft is needed. If so, and if autograft is indicated, then the iliac crest provides a readily available source of cortico-cancellous graft. Alternatively, structural allograft may be combined with cancellous autograft or bone marrow aspirate.

The final question is whether there is a need for the enhanced biology associated with iliac crest graft. The authors routinely use some form of iliac crest graft in smokers, diabetics, patients with a history of substantial soft-tissue stripping, and patients undergoing revision fusion.

Contraindications to autograft include grafting into a site with active infection or one in which infection is likely to occur such as open injuries and fractures with bone loss. In these cases, the contaminated tissue must be debrided and the infection cleared before bone grafting. Other relative contraindications include prior surgeries performed at the site of planned bone graft harvest and compromised skin from burns, scars, or other trauma. For the iliac crest in particular, morbid obesity is a relative contraindication if the incision falls within a skin fold or under a pannus. Contraindications to harvesting around the knee or from the intramedullary canal (RIA) would be the presence of a prosthesis or hardware from fracture fixation, especially an intramedullary nail. Osteoporosis is another relative contraindication for RIA.[27]

SURGICAL TECHNIQUE
Preoperative Planning

Depending on the type of bone graft to be harvested, appropriate instruments should be readily available. For harvest at the iliac crest, tibia, or calcaneus, most instruments are found in a standard foot and ankle instrument set. Special instruments may include trephines, saws, burrs, or various gouges and curettes that can be used to create a corticotomy in the bone and extract the graft.

Also, if planning to obtain graft using the reamer-irrigator-aspirator, the surgeon needs to request appropriate guide wires and reamers. Knowing the exact diameter of the isthmus of the femur or tibia may decrease complications associated with the RIA, including incarceration of the reamer head or iatrogenic fracture.[24] When using the RIA for graft harvest, the authors initially do not ream past the isthmus. Once the bone graft is harvested, the volume is assessed, and if more graft is needed, we then ream past the isthmus after widening the canal with standard flexible reamers.

Preparation and Patient Positioning

Bone graft harvest, regardless of location, is invariability a secondary procedure. As such, the patient positioning should maximize ease and exposure for the primary surgery. Depending on positioning, this may preclude bone graft harvest from specific areas. For example, if a prone position is needed for a posterior ankle fusion, the patient would not be properly positioned for an anterior iliac crest graft harvest. However, a calcaneal graft would still be possible. The major factor for preparation and positioning is that the surgeon retains access to the donor site and plans skin preparation and draping appropriately.

Specific to the iliac crest, it is often useful to position the patient with a bump under the ipsilateral hip. This method may also facilitate the index procedure being performed distally. The bump will allow the patient's soft tissue to fall away and leave the crest more palpable. Similarly, for patients with a protuberant abdomen, it can be useful to retract the pannus with broad tape to hold it away and allow easier access to the crest.

When considering using the RIA, the approach must be carefully planned as well. The authors often use a retrograde approach as described below. With most RIA procedures, the patient is positioned prone. The extremity must simply be prepared and draped further proximally based on the harvest site.

Iliac Crest Bone Graft

The anterior iliac crest can be used to obtain simple bone marrow aspirate or to openly harvest cancellous and cortico-cancellous grafts. As noted, the average maximal bone graft that can be obtained from the anterior iliac crest is approximately 20 cm^3.[4] More may be obtained from the posterior crest, but this is rarely used in foot and ankle surgery because of patient positioning. The bone is harvested from the adjacent iliac tubercle approximately 3 to 5 cm posterior to the anterior superior iliac spine to avoid injury to the lateral femoral cutaneous nerve.

Surgical procedure

1. An incision is made parallel to the iliac crest and approximately 3 to 5 cm posterior to the anterior superior iliac spine.
2. The lateral femoral cutaneous nerve is protected in the anterior extent of the incision.
3. Subperiosteal dissection is performed with electro cautery to the level of the iliac crest.
4. The iliacus muscle is elevated from the inner table and the gluteus medius from the outer table if exposure is needed for a cortico-cancellous bone graft.

Cancellous bone graft

5. The cortex from the superior iliac crest is removed using a burr or osteotome.
6. Either a trap door or oval window is created in the superior crest. A round or oval window minimizes stress risers.
7. Cancellous graft is harvested with a curette or gauge.
8. If more than 10 cm^0 is removed, the surgeon should consider filling the resulting void with allograft.

Tricortical bone graft

9. Full subperiosteal dissection of the crest is completed as above.
10. The desired length of bone is measured along the rim and the bone cuts marked with electrocautery.
11. The proximal and distal cuts are made with an osteotome or microsagittal saw to the desired depth.
12. The lateral musculature is reflected to allow a visualization of the outer table.
13. The soft tissues medial to the inner table are protected with a lap pad or retractor placed between the inner table and iliacus muscle.
14. The transverse cut is then made using an osteotome or sagittal saw to complete the harvest.

Closure

15. The wound is closed in layers including periosteum, fascia, subcutaneous tissue, and skin. With meticulous hemostasis, drains are rarely necessary.

Proximal Tibial Bone Graft

In the authors' experience, the proximal tibia is favored over the distal tibia. The rational for this is the volume of graft necessary and to preserve regional anatomy and bone stock about the ankle.

Surgical procedure

1. A 2- to 3-cm oblique incision is made overlying Gerdy's tubercle (**Fig. 2**).
2. The fascia of the anterior compartment and iliotibial band is incised along its fibers.
3. Gerdy's tubercle and additional cortex are exposed as needed in a subperiosteal fashion. A burr is used to make an oval window in the cortex.
4. The cancellous bone graft is then harvested with a curette.

Distal Tibial Bone Graft

The authors consider distal tibial graft when the primary surgery is isolated to the hind-foot, midfoot, or forefoot.

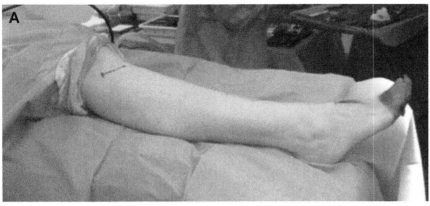

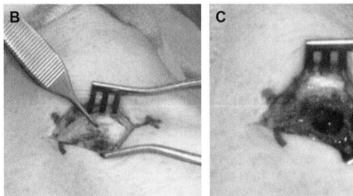

Fig. 2. (*A*) Proximal tibial incision. (*B*) Dissection to the cortex. (*C*) Round corticotomy and curettage to remove bone graft.

Surgical procedure

1. A 2- to 3-cm incision is made along the medial aspect of the distal tibia at the metaphysical flare.
2. The saphenous vein and nerve, which are often visualized in the field, must be protected.
3. A corticotomy is then made using a burr or trephine.
4. If a trephine is used, it may be passed to the lateral cortex under hand power to obtain a dowel of cancellous bone graft. The far cortex should not be perforated.
5. Fluoroscopy is used to confirm that the corticotomy is centered on the bone and that the joint is not violated.
6. A curette is used to harvest additional bone through the corticotomy until sufficient graft has been obtained.

Calcaneal Bone Graft

Calcaneal autograft is generally used for procedures in midfoot and forefoot.

Surgical procedure

1. An oblique 1- to 1.5-cm incision is made along the lateral calcaneus approximately 2 cm anterior to the calcaneal tuberosity and 2 cm superior to the plantar foot (**Fig. 3**).

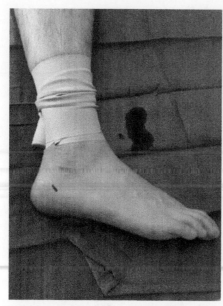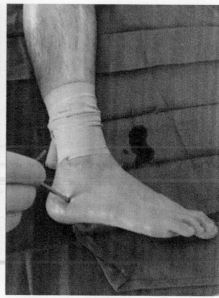

Fig. 3. Calcaneal bone graft harvested with a trephine.

2. Blunt dissection is used to expose the lateral wall of the calcaneus. The sural nerve and its branches are at risk during this step of the procedure and must be protected.
3. The periosteum is elevated with a freer elevator.
4. A 7- to 8-mm trephine is used to perforate the lateral wall under hand power and then passed up to the medial wall of the tuberosity. This method harvests a unicortical dowel of cancellous bone. If the medial wall is also perforated, a bicortical dowel may also be removed.
5. Additional graft may be harvested with a trephine or curette through the initial corticotomy.

Reamer-Irrigator-Aspirator Harvest

There are multiple techniques for accessing the intramedullary canal of the femur and tibia. When considering a tibio-talar-calcaneal fusion with a nail, the RIA may be used through the same plantar incision as the fusion nail itself.[28] For an antegrade approach to the tibia or femur, the initial exposure is identical to that used for inserting a standard intramedullary nail. The exception is for a retrograde approach to the femur. Some have described access via the intracondylar notch, but this approach necessitates an arthrotomy.[7,29] An alternative is to use a lateral condylar entry point similar to the entry point used for flexible intramedullary nails in pediatric fracture fixation.

Surgical procedure

1. A 3-cm vertical incision is made half way between lateral trochlea and the lateral epicondyle.
2. The fascia of the iliotibial band is incised in line with the fibers.

3. The lateral collateral ligament, inserting on the lateral epicondyle, should be protected.
4. A burr is used to open the cortex and facilitate passage of the guide wire into the canal.
5. A reamer is then used to widen the entry point for the RIA. The smallest RIA cutting head is 12 mm diameter
6. Before reaming, ensure that the device is properly connected and that the trap is connected, otherwise the graft can be suctioned into the waste container.
7. The isthmus should be measured preoperatively to ensure safe passage of the reamer.
8. The canal proximal to the isthmus may be reamed without crossing the isthmus depending on the quantity of graft required.
9. Once the 12-mm reamer has passed, the head size may be increased and progressively widened to obtain more graft.
10. When the reamer is not in use, the suction must be turned off avoid increased blood loss.
11. Closure should be in layers including periosteum and fascia.

COMPLICATIONS

Minor and major complications after autograft harvest are well described in the literature.[3,8,10,11,13,30] Minor complications include those that do not cause long-term disability or substantially alter the treatment course. Examples include sensory nerve injury, seroma, superficial infections, or mild donor site pain. Major complications include those that require additional intervention or cause substantial morbidity, such as deep infections or hematoma, major neurovascular injury, or fracture.

Iliac Crest

Younger and Chapman[11] were one of the first to draw attention to the potential for high complication rates with iliac crest graft. In their study of 243 iliac crest harvests, they noted a 20.6% minor complication rate. Of note, the grafts were harvested primarily for spine and trauma. The authors also reported an 8.6% major complication rate, including deep infection (2.5%), reoperation (3.8%), large hematoma (3.3%), and pain lasting longer than 6 months (2.5%).[11] Similar results were found in another study of 414 iliac crest harvests that reported a 10% rate of minor and a 5.8% risk of major complications including iliac wing fractures, vascular injury, and deep infections.[8] Specific to the iliac crest, if a large cortico-cancellous segment of the crest is harvested, concern for incisional hernia and gait disturbance caused by detaching the gluteus medius is described.[8]

In the foot and ankle, complication rates are generally lower. DeOrio and Farber[5] published a series of 134 patients after iliac crest graft harvest used for foot and ankle procedures. They reported a 90% satisfaction with the procedure and a low rate of complications including a 6.7% incidence of hematoma. Only 10% of patients had lasting pain at the harvest site. There were no deep infections. Another study described using tricortical graft for fusion after failed total ankle arthrodesis and reported no infections and only 1 nonunion out of 16 patients.[3]

Of note, early pain is common after iliac crest harvest, and the patient should be counseled that this is most often temporary and will resolve after several months. In the authors' experience, it can be minimized by not stripping the inner and outer tables of the crest, if possible.

Proximal Tibia

Proximal tibia bone grafts used for foot and ankle procedures have low complication rates.[20,31] In one study, there were no major complications, and only 1 of 54 patients sustained a local hematoma. There were no fractures.[31] O'Keeffe and colleagues[20] reported on 230 proximal tibial harvests and noted a 1.3% complication rate and safe resumption of weight bearing within 6 weeks. One study found higher rates of minor complications including superficial hematomas in 15% of patients.[32] The graft harvests, however, were performed as an adjunct for head and neck procedures. It should also be noted that this study was reported in the nonorthopedic literature and may have been performed by surgeons not as familiar with extremity anatomy.

Major complications have been reported infrequently but can include proximal joint perforation, deep hematoma, and gait disturbances and fracture. All of these were reported to occur in less than 2% of patients.[20,31–34]

Calcaneus

After calcaneal bone graft harvest, Raikin and Brislin[19] reported that 5 of 44 patients had persistent pain with shoe wear. All symptoms, however, resolved within 6 months with desensitization therapy. Two patients did have decreased sensation in the sural nerve distribution, but this did not affect function. O'Malley and colleagues[30] evaluated 393 patients who underwent a calcaneal graft harvest. A total of 86.2% of patients reported no donor site pain. Only 6 patients (2.9%) reported sural nerve sensitivity, whereas 4 patients (1.9%) noted incision pain, and another 4 (1.9%) noted transient incisional numbness. Three patients (1.4%) had major complications, including a fracture through the graft site, a stress fracture, and permanent numbness in the sural nerve. Overall, there was a 13.8% incidence of minor symptoms after graft harvest despite the relative ease of the procedure. However, most of these did not have any significant long-term impact.[30]

Reamer-Irrigator-Aspirator

In a study by Lowe and colleagues,[27] 6 complications were reported out of 97 RIA harvest procedures (6.2%). These complications included 4 fractures, all of which occurred in the postoperative setting. Other studies reported reamer becoming incarcerated when attempting to over-ream the isthmus by greater than 2 mm.[24,35] Finally, blood loss may be a concern with RIA. One study reported blood loss as high as 500 mL.[35] This same study reported a case in which the reamer was lodged in the bone for 3 minutes with the suction active, resulting in a substantial blood loss that required transfusion. With regard to minor complications, Belthur and colleagues[25] reported on 41 patients undergoing RIA with 2 complications: 1 patient with eccentric reaming and femoral cortex perforation and another who had an impending femoral neck fracture and required prophylactic screw fixation. They also reported lower pain scores and no other donor site complications compared with iliac crest harvest.[25]

Proper assembly of the RIA along with appropriate selection of the reamer head not to exceed 1.5 to 2 mm greater than the isthmus of the femur or tibia will decrease the chance of the most catastrophic complications, such as fracture or substantial blood loss. Careful use of the fluoroscopy is also advised. The technique, although familiar to many surgeons who perform long bone intramedullary fixation, is still sufficiently different that experts have recommended specific training before first use in clinical practice.[24,35,36]

POSTOPERATIVE CARE

In general, postoperative weight bearing is dictated by the limitations imposed by the index procedure. If the same dressing as the primary procedure is used, then no change in wound care instructions to cover the harvest site are necessary. If the harvest site has a separate dressing, the patient is typically advised to leave this in place until the first postoperative visit.

Most of the grafts harvested for foot and ankle surgeries are small and do not present a structural problem for weight bearing. Possible exceptions would be if a large quantity of proximal tibial graft were harvested. However, in this instance, it would generally be used for a procedure that would likely mandate non–weight bearing or limited weight bearing as well.

Finally, when an RIA technique is used with an entry point near the knee, the patient should be given a knee immobilizer for the first several days or until the first postoperative visit facilitate wound healing. Thereafter, the patients are encouraged to regularly range the knee through its full arc of motion to prevent stiffness. Typically, no muscle is divided during this approach; therefore, knee weakness is not an issue for patients after recovery.

SUMMARY

Foot and ankle surgeons have several options when it comes to harvesting autologous bone graft. The iliac crest has been the common donor site and is still frequently used. However, sufficient bone may also be expeditiously harvested from the proximal and distal tibial metaphyses, the calcaneus, and the intramedullary canals of both the tibia and femur.

The decision as to which harvest site to use is made on a case-by-case basis and depends on several factors. These factors include anatomic proximity, the volume of graft desired, the need for structural graft, and the intrinsic biology of the particular donor site. Most autograft can be obtained safely and reliably with minimal increase in operating time. Nevertheless, patients should be appropriately counseled about the risks and potential complications, including donor site pain, of the graft the surgeon plans on using. Fortunately, most complications are minor and do not cause long-term morbidity.

REFERENCES

1. Ahlmann E, Patzakis M, Roidis N, et al. Comparison of anterior and posterior iliac crest bone grafts in terms of harvest-site morbidity and functional outcomes. J Bone Joint Surg Am 2002;84-A:716–20.

2. Bhosale A, Munoruth A, Blundell C, et al. Complex primary arthrodesis of the first metatarsophalangeal joint after bone loss. Foot Ankle Int 2011;32:968–72.

3. Culpan P, Le Strat V, Piriou P, et al. Arthrodesis after failed total ankle replacement. J Bone Joint Surg Br 2007;89:1178–83.

4. Dawson J, Kiner D, Gardner W 2nd, et al. The reamer-irrigator-aspirator as a device for harvesting bone graft compared with iliac crest bone graft: union rates and complications. J Orthop Trauma 2014;28:584–90.

5. DeOrio JK, Farber DC. Morbidity associated with anterior iliac crest bone grafting in foot and ankle surgery. Foot Ankle Int 2005;26:147–51.

6. Khan SN, Cammisa FP Jr, Sandhu HS, et al. The biology of bone grafting. J Am Acad Orthop Surg 2005;13:77–86.

7. Myeroff C, Archdeacon M. Autogenous bone graft: donor sites and techniques. J Bone Joint Surg Am 2011;93:2227–36.

8. Arrington ED, Smith WJ, Chambers HG, et al. Complications of iliac crest bone graft harvesting. Clin Orthop Relat Res 1996;(329):300–9.

9. Banwart JC, Asher MA, Hassanein RS. Iliac crest bone graft harvest donor site morbidity. A statistical evaluation. Spine (Phila Pa 1976) 1995;20:1055–60.

10. Goulet JA, Senunas LE, DeSilva GL, et al. Autogenous iliac crest bone graft. Complications and functional assessment. Clin Orthop Relat Res 1997;(339): 76–81.

11. Younger EM, Chapman MW. Morbidity at bone graft donor sites. J Orthop Trauma 1989;3:192–5.

12. Allsopp BJ, Hunter-Smith DJ, Rozen WM. Vascularized versus nonvascularized bone grafts: what is the evidence? Clin Orthop Relat Res 2016;474:1319–27.

13. Fishman FG, Adams SB, Easley ME, et al. Vascularized pedicle bone grafting for nonunions of the tarsal navicular. Foot Ankle Int 2012;33:734–9.

14. Chiodo CP, Hahne J, Wilson MG, et al. Histological differences in iliac and tibial bone graft. Foot Ankle Int 2010;31:418–22.

15. Hyer CF, Berlet GC, Bussewitz BW, et al. Quantitative assessment of the yield of osteoblastic connective tissue progenitors in bone marrow aspirate from the iliac crest, tibia, and calcaneus. J Bone Joint Surg Am 2013;95:1312–6.

16. Grier KM, Walling AK. The use of tricortical autograft versus allograft in lateral column lengthening for adult acquired flatfoot deformity: an analysis of union rates and complications. Foot Ankle Int 2010;31:760–9.

17. Herford AS, King BJ, Audia F, et al. Medial approach for tibial bone graft: anatomic study and clinical technique. J Oral Maxillofac Surg 2003;61:358–63.

18. van Damme PA, Merkx MA. A modification of the tibial bone-graft-harvesting technique. Int J Oral Maxillofac Surg 1996;25:346–8.

19. Raikin SM, Brislin K. Local bone graft harvested from the distal tibia or calcaneus for surgery of the foot and ankle. Foot Ankle Int 2005;26:449–53.

20. O'Keeffe RM Jr, Riemer BL, Butterfield SL. Harvesting of autogenous cancellous bone graft from the proximal tibial metaphysis. A review of 230 cases. J Orthop Trauma 1991;5:469–74.

21. Biddinger KR, Komenda GA, Schon LC, et al. A new modified technique for harvest of calcaneal bone grafts in surgery on the foot and ankle. Foot Ankle Int 1998;19:322–6.

22. Roukis T. A simple technique for harvesting autogenous bone grafts from the calcaneus. Foot Ankle Int 2006;27:998–9.

23. DiDomenico LA, Haro AA 3rd. Percutaneous harvest of calcaneal bone graft. J Foot Ankle Surg 2006;45:131–3.

24. Masquelet AC, Benko PE, Mathevon H, et al. Harvest of cortico-cancellous intramedullary femoral bone graft using the Reamer-Irrigator-Aspirator (RIA). Orthop Traumatol Surg Res 2012;98:227–32.

25. Belthur MV, Conway JD, Jindal G, et al. Bone graft harvest using a new intramedullary system. Clin Orthop Relat Res 2008;466:2973–80.

26. Sagi HC, Young ML, Gerstenfeld L, et al. Qualitative and quantitative differences between bone graft obtained from the medullary canal (with a Reamer/Irrigator/Aspirator) and the iliac crest of the same patient. J Bone Joint Surg Am 2012; 94:2128–35.

27. Lowe JA, Della Rocca GJ, Murtha Y, et al. Complications associated with negative pressure reaming for harvesting autologous bone graft: a case series. J Orthop Trauma 2010;24:46–52.

28. Herscovici D Jr, Scaduto JM. Use of the reamer-irrigator-aspirator technique to obtain autograft for ankle and hindfoot arthrodesis. J Bone Joint Surg Br 2012; 94:75–9.
29. Mansour J, Conway JD. Retrograde reamer/irrigator/aspirator technique for autologous bone graft harvesting with the patient in the prone position. Am J Orthop (Belle Mead NJ) 2015;44:202–5.
30. O'Malley MJ, Sayres SC, Saleem O, et al. Morbidity and complications following percutaneous calcaneal autograft bone harvest. Foot Ankle Int 2014;35:30–7.
31. Alt V, Nawab A, Seligson D. Bone grafting from the proximal tibia. J Trauma 1999; 47:555–7.
32. Chen YC, Chen CH, Chen PL, et al. Donor site morbidity after harvesting of proximal tibia bone. Head Neck 2006;28:496–500.
33. Galano GJ, Greisberg JK. Tibial plateau fracture with proximal tibia autograft harvest for foot surgery. Am J Orthop (Belle Mead NJ) 2009;38:621–3.
34. Geideman W, Early JS, Brodsky J. Clinical results of harvesting autogenous cancellous graft from the ipsilateral proximal tibia for use in foot and ankle surgery. Foot Ankle Int 2004;25:451–5.
35. Quintero AJ, Tarkin IS, Pape HC. Technical tricks when using the reamer irrigator aspirator technique for autologous bone graft harvesting. J Orthop Trauma 2010; 24:42–5.
36. Giannoudis PV, Tzioupis C, Green J. Surgical techniques: how I do it? The Reamer/Irrigator/Aspirator (RIA) system. Injury 2009;40:1231–6.

Bone Marrow Aspirate Concentrate for Bone Healing in Foot and Ankle Surgery

Joshua S. Harford, MS, Travis J. Dekker, MD,
Samuel B. Adams, MD*

KEYWORDS

- Bone marrow aspirate • Concentrate • BMAC • Cartilage • Bone

KEY POINTS

- Bone marrow aspirate concentrate (BMAC) contains mesenchymal stem cells, hematopoietic stem cells, other progenitor cells, bone morphogenetic proteins, and growth factors essential for bone healing.
- Strong animal evidence exists to support the use of BMAC for bone healing.
- Human data on the use of BMAC are promising but lack scientific rigor to validate its efficacy.

INTRODUCTION

Arthrodesis remains the gold standard treatment of end-stage arthritis of the joints of the foot and ankle. Unfortunately, many patients have comorbidities that portend to an increase risk of nonunion, including smoking, diabetes, and avascular necrosis, among others. In various ways, all of these comorbidities compromise vascularity and, in turn, the delivery of nutrients and host reparative cells to the arthrodesis site. Attempting arthrodesis in these high-risk patients has led to nonunion rates as high as 40%, which can lead to persistent pain and debilitation.[1–4] Therefore, a need exists to find adjuncts to achieve union in foot and ankle arthrodesis procedures.

Autologous bone marrow aspirate concentrate (BMAC) has been successfully used for bone and soft-tissue healing.[5–8] The proposed benefit is the collection and transplantation of live cells and growth factors. BMAC contains mesenchymal stem cells (MSCs), hematopoietic stem cells (HSCs), endothelial progenitor cells, and other progenitor cells, in addition to growth factors, including bone morphogenetic proteins,

The authors have nothing to disclose.
Department of Orthopaedic Surgery, Duke University Medical Center, Durham, NC 27710, USA
* Corresponding author. Department of Orthopaedic Surgery, Duke University Medical Center, 4709 Creekstone Drive, Durham, NC 27703.
E-mail address: samuel.adams@duke.edu

Foot Ankle Clin N Am 21 (2016) 839–845
http://dx.doi.org/10.1016/j.fcl.2016.07.005
1083-7515/16/© 2016 Elsevier Inc. All rights reserved.

platelet-derived growth factor, transforming growth factor-β, vascular endothelial growth factor, interleukin-8, and interleukin-1 receptor antagonist. It must be noted that the term *MSC* is not universally accepted and some investigators favor connective tissue progenitors (CTPs) or mesenchymal stromal cells (also MSCs).

Although unconcentrated bone marrow aspirate contains all of these same elements, concentration has been shown to significantly improve healing because a theoretic critical number of certain cellular elements, rather than the total cell count, has been shown to be more important.[9,10] Moreover, in foot and ankle surgeries, limited amounts of physical space exist for biologics implantation; therefore, concentration may be beneficial.

Both the MSCs and HSCs have the potential to differentiate into osteogenic progenitors. This differentiation can occur with the assistance of growth factors and induction proteins either locally (where the BMAC is transplanted to) or through these agents that are contained within the BMAC. Moreover, these cells have a paracrine effect to recruit additional host cells to the delivery site and enhance additional growth factor protein production in paracrine fashion.

Despite the theoretic advantages of BMAC, the level 1 clinical evidence for its use is minimal. In this article, the authors review the orthopedic literature and, more specifically, the foot and ankle literature for the use of BMAC for bone healing.

ANIMAL EVIDENCE

Several animal studies exist demonstrating solid evidence for its use in aiding bone healing. Gianakos and colleagues[11] performed a review of all of the available evidence regarding long-bone healing in animals. They found overwhelmingly positive evidence for BMAC, with more than 35 articles included in that review. Of the studies reporting statistics, 100% showed a significant increase in bone formation in the BMAC groups compared with controls. Radiographic and micro–computed tomography (CT) imaging from these studies demonstrated a significant increase in bone volume, callus formation, woven bone formation, and union. Histology studies corroborated radiographic findings of significant or semiquantitative improvement in osteocyte number and bone formation.

However, the evidence is not always positive in favor of BMAC and seems to be less promising in metaphyseal defects. In a study of tibial metaphyseal bone healing in mini-pigs, Jungbluth and colleagues[12] compared the use of autograft, BMAC, and calcium phosphate. The BMAC group demonstrated significantly more bone formation compared with the calcium phosphate group, but the autograft group demonstrated significantly more bone formation than the BMAC group. Another study compared BMAC with platelet-rich plasma (PRP) on metaphyseal defects in rabbit tibiae.[13] CT and histomorphometry data demonstrated greater cortical bone and greater consolidation in the PRP group at 4 weeks.

CLINICAL REPORTS
Non–Foot and Ankle Studies

Several studies are reported describing use of BMAC for bone healing outside of the foot and ankle. Most of these studies have focused on osteonecrosis of the femoral head or tibia fracture nonunions.

Pepke and colleagues[14] performed a prospective randomized trial of 24 patients with osteonecrosis of the femoral head. Patients were randomized to core decompression only versus core decompression and BMAC. All patients were followed for 2 years after surgery. There was no significant difference in clinical outcome or femoral head survival. Similarly, another study retrospectively reviewed 60 hips in 45 patients with osteonecrosis of the femoral head.[15] Nineteen hips were treated with core decompression alone, and 41 hips were treated with core decompression plus BMAC. Postoperatively, there was no difference in the incidence of head collapse.

The popularity of BMAC increased after its use for tibial shaft nonunions. Hernigou and colleagues[9] reported on the use of percutaneous BMAC injections to 60 atrophic nonunions of the tibia. They were able to achieve union in 53 patients. Interestingly, the 7 patients that continued to have a nonunion received a significantly lower total number and concentration of progenitor cells, implying a theoretic critical number.

Foot and Ankle–Specific Studies

Few reports exist describing the use BMAC in foot and ankle surgery. Murawski and Kennedy[16] performed percutaneous screw fixation plus BMAC for proximal fifth metatarsal (Jones type) fractures in 26 athletic patients. At a mean follow-up of 21 months, 24 of these patients achieved union without complication at a mean of 5 weeks after surgery. One patient experienced delayed union and one patient healed but refractured. Overall, this patient population experienced significant improvement in the Foot and Ankle Outcome Score and both the physical and mental components of the 12-Item Short Form Survey. Similarly, O'Malley and colleagues[17] retrospectively reviewed the charts of 10 National Basketball Association players with Jones fractures treated with internal fixation and BMAC. They noted a mean time to fracture healing of 7.5 weeks. Three patients refractured. Unfortunately, both of these studies lack a control group; it is, therefore, difficult to assess the benefit of BMAC in bone healing of the foot and ankle.

In a retrospective case-control study of diabetic patients with ankle fracture nonunions, Hernigou and colleagues[18] compared 86 patients who received BMAC injection with 86 historically matched diabetic patients who received iliac crest bone graft for the treatment of the ankle fracture nonunions. Seventy (82%) of the 86 diabetic patients treated with BMAC demonstrated healing, whereas only 53 (62%) of the 86 diabetic patients who received iliac crest bone graft demonstrated healing. These findings were significant in favor of the BMAC group. Moreover, the iliac crest harvest group had a significantly higher rate of major and minor complications.

Finally, Adams and colleagues[19] delivered BMAC through a percutaneous cannulated screw to treat a stress fracture of the medial cuneiform. The stress fracture had failed conservative management. The cannula in the screw was covered with wax, and the BMAC was successfully injected by inserting the needle through the wax down the screw cannula into the medial cuneiform. Stress fracture union was confirmed with postoperative CT.

SAFETY

In addition to the aforementioned foot and ankle–specific studies, several additional studies have described the safety of BMAC in orthopedic conditions. One of the most concerning potential problems with delivering MSCs into a new location is the potential for tumorigenesis. However, this theory is unfounded in at least one large series. This series retrospectively reviewed the charts and images of 1873 patients treated with BMAC at a mean follow-up of 12.5 years.[20] More than 7300 MRIs and 52,000 radiographs were reviewed. Fifty-three cancers were diagnosed in areas other than the BMAC injection site. However, from the cancer incidence in the general population, the expected cancer incidence over the same study time period was theoretically between 97 and 108.

MAXIMIZING EFFICACY

Several investigators have investigated ways to maximize the concentration of stem cells from bone marrow aspirate. There are several centrifugation machines for bone marrow aspirate concentration, all with different, mostly proprietary, methods of marrow processing and centrifugation settings. Hegde and colleagues[21] performed a direct comparison of 3 different clinically available centrifugation systems (Harvest SmartPreP 2, Harvest Terumo BCT, Lakewood, CO; Biomet BioCUE, Zimmer-Biomet, Warsaw, IN; Arteriocyte Magellan; Arteriocyte Medical Systems, Cleveland, OH). The Harvest system was compared with both the Biomet and the Arteriocyte systems in 2 separate arms of the study. For each patient, each anterior iliac crest was randomized to have the Harvest and one other system for bilateral iliac crest aspiration. The Harvest system achieved a significantly greater number and concentration of CTPs both before and after centrifugation compared with the Zimmer-Biomet system. The Harvest system also demonstrated a significantly greater number and concentration of CTPs after centrifugation compared with the Arteriocyte system. Because of the positive results of the Harvest system, the Zimmer-Biomet and Arteriocyte systems were never directly compared.

The location of aspiration is also important. Typical locations for bone marrow aspiration include the posterior iliac crest, the anterior iliac crest, the proximal tibia, the distal tibia, and the calcaneus. Obviously, the distal tibia and calcaneus are the most convenient for foot and ankle surgeries because they are included in the sterile field, but evidence has demonstrated that they do not contain the most robust cell population. Review of the literature has demonstrated that the quantity of osteogenic progenitor cells decreases from the axial to appendicular skeleton as well as from proximal to distal in the appendicular skeleton. In fact, vertebral bodies were found to have a higher quantity of osteogenic progenitor cells than in control-matched iliac crests.[22] However, aspiration from the vertebral bodies in nonspine surgery is not realistic. However, the iliac crest is a good source of osteogenic progenitor cells. Hyer and colleagues[23] demonstrated that the anterior iliac crest contained a significantly higher mean concentration of osteogenic progenitor cells when compared with the distal tibia and calcaneus in the same patient. There was no significant difference between the distal tibia and the calcaneus. They also demonstrated no difference in cell yield with increased age, sex, smoking, and diabetes, all factors thought to decrease the osteoprogenitor cell population in bone marrow and increase the risk of nonunion in foot and ankle arthrodesis procedures. Moreover, Pierini and colleagues[24] demonstrated that the posterior iliac crest contained, on average, 1.6 times more progenitor cells. However, Marx and Tursun[25] demonstrated that the cell yield from the anterior and posterior iliac crest was the same but twice as much as that obtained from the proximal tibia. Therefore, the authors recommend aspiration from the anterior iliac crest during surgery when patients are supine and from the posterior iliac crest when patients are prone.

The technique of aspiration is also important to cell yield. Rapid aspiration of large volumes at once is thought to create peripheral blood dilution of the bone marrow. Although this saves operative time, it has been shown to reduce progenitor cell yield. Hernigou and colleagues[26] compared the use of 10- and 50-mL syringes.

Despite the larger volume of the 50-mL syringe, they demonstrated an average of 300% higher cell yield with the 10-mL syringe. Moreover, this same study demonstrated significantly more cells in the first 1 mL aspirate of the 10-mL syringe compared with the first 5 mL of the 50-mL syringe. This study demonstrated that better cell yield could be obtained by aspirating small volumes in small syringes.

CASE EXAMPLE

The patient is a 54-year-old man who had previous lateralizing calcaneus osteotomy for hindfoot varus. He complained of heel pain. Radiographs demonstrated a nonunion and malposition of his calcaneus osteotomy (**Fig. 1**A). He failed conservative management and elected to undergo revision surgery. At the time of surgery, he underwent hardware removal, debridement, and reduction of his calcaneal tuberosity. Ipsilateral iliac crest bone marrow aspirate was obtained and concentrated. The guidewires for the calcaneus screws were placed and the lateral incision was closed. Next, the guidewires were sequentially overdrilled for the screws. The screws were placed up to the level of the nonunion site. Bone wax was placed in the screw cannulation at the head. Next, the concentrated bone marrow aspirate was injected through the wax and into the nonunion site as previously described (**Fig. 1**B).[19] Postoperative CT scan demonstrates a healed calcaneus osteotomy site at 4 months after revision surgery (**Fig. 1**C, D).

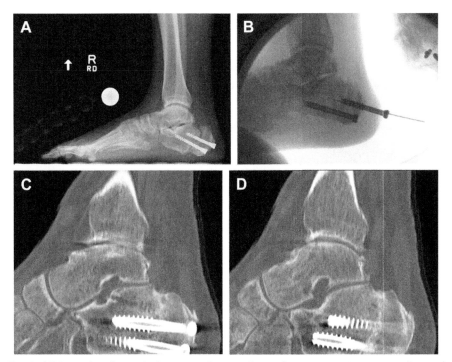

Fig. 1. (A) Lateral radiograph demonstrating previous calcaneus osteotomy nonunion and malposition. (B) Intraoperative fluoroscopy demonstrating concentrated bone marrow aspirate injection through the screw cannulation into the nonunion site. (C, D) Sagittal CT scan images demonstrating union of the osteotomy site.

SUMMARY

Most animal studies demonstrate promising results for the use of autologous BMAC on bone healing. Although the literature on the use of BMAC in the foot and ankle is promising, further prospective and/or comparative studies are needed. BMAC should be considered in patients with traditional risk factors for nonunion.

REFERENCES

1. DiGiovanni CW, Lin SS, Baumhauer JF, et al. Recombinant human platelet-derived growth factor-BB and beta-tricalcium phosphate (rhPDGF-BB/beta-TCP): an alternative to autogenous bone graft. J Bone Joint Surg Am 2013; 95(13):1184–92.
2. Frey C, Halikus NM, Vu-Rose T, et al. A review of ankle arthrodesis: predisposing factors to nonunion. Foot Ankle Int 1994;15(11):581–4.
3. Easley ME, Trnka HJ, Schon LC, et al. Isolated subtalar arthrodesis. J Bone Joint Surg Am 2000;82(5):613–24.
4. O'Connor KM, Johnson JE, McCormick JJ, et al. Clinical and operative factors related to successful revision arthrodesis in the foot and ankle. Foot Ankle Int 2016;37(8):809–15.
5. Adams SB Jr, Thorpe MA, Parks BG, et al. Stem cell-bearing suture improves Achilles tendon healing in a rat model. Foot Ankle Int 2014;35(3):293–9.
6. Connolly JF, Guse R, Tiedeman J, et al. Autologous marrow injection as a substitute for operative grafting of tibial nonunions. Clin Orthop Relat Res 1991;266: 259–70.
7. Fortier LA, Potter HG, Rickey EJ, et al. Concentrated bone marrow aspirate improves full-thickness cartilage repair compared with microfracture in the equine model. J Bone Joint Surg Am 2010;92(10):1927–37.
8. Gangji V, De Maertelaer V, Hauzeur JP. Autologous bone marrow cell implantation in the treatment of non-traumatic osteonecrosis of the femoral head: five year follow-up of a prospective controlled study. Bone 2011;49(5):1005–9.
9. Hernigou P, Poignard A, Beaujean F. Percutaneous autologous bone-marrow grafting for nonunions. Influence of the number and concentration of progenitor cells. J Bone Joint Surg Am 2005;87(7):1430–7.
10. Connolly J, Guse R, Lippiello L, et al. Development of an osteogenic bone-marrow preparation. J Bone Joint Surg Am 1989;71(5):684–91.
11. Gianakos A, Ni A, Zambrana L, et al. Bone marrow aspirate concentrate in animal long bone healing: an analysis of basic science evidence. J Orthop Trauma 2016; 30(1):1–9.
12. Jungbluth P, Hakimi AR, Grassmann JP, et al. The early phase influence of bone marrow concentrate on metaphyseal bone healing. Injury 2013;44(10):1285–94.
13. Batista MA, Leivas TP, Rodrigues CJ, et al. Comparison between the effects of platelet-rich plasma and bone marrow concentrate on defect consolidation in the rabbit tibia. Clinics (Sao Paulo) 2011;66(10):1787–92.
14. Pepke W, Kasten P, Beckmann NA, et al. Core decompression and autologous bone marrow concentrate for treatment of femoral head osteonecrosis: a randomized prospective study. Orthop Rev (Pavia) 2016;8(1):6162.
15. Cruz-Pardos A, Garcia-Rey E, Ortega-Chamarro JA, et al. Mid-term comparative outcomes of autologous bone-marrow concentration to treat osteonecrosis of the femoral head in standard practice. Hip Int 2016. [Epub ahead of print].
16. Murawski CD, Kennedy JG. Percutaneous internal fixation of proximal fifth metatarsal jones fractures (zones II and III) with Charlotte Carolina screw and bone

marrow aspirate concentrate: an outcome study in athletes. Am J Sports Med 2011;39(6):1295–301.

17. O'Malley M, DeSandis B, Allen A, et al. Operative treatment of fifth metatarsal jones fractures (zones II and III) in the NBA. Foot Ankle Int 2016;37(5):488–500.

18. Hernigou P, Guissou I, Homma Y, et al. Percutaneous injection of bone marrow mesenchymal stem cells for ankle non-unions decreases complications in patients with diabetes. Int Orthop 2015;39(8):1639–43.

19. Adams SB, Lewis JS Jr, Gupta AK, et al. Cannulated screw delivery of bone marrow aspirate concentrate to a stress fracture nonunion: technique tip. Foot Ankle Int 2013;34(5):740–4.

20. Hernigou P, Homma Y, Flouzat-Lachaniette CH, et al. Cancer risk is not increased in patients treated for orthopaedic diseases with autologous bone marrow cell concentrate. J Bone Joint Surg Am 2013;95(24):2215–21.

21. Hegde V, Shonuga O, Ellis S, et al. A prospective comparison of 3 approved systems for autologous bone marrow concentration demonstrated nonequivalency in progenitor cell number and concentration. J Orthop Trauma 2014;28(10):591–8.

22. McLain RF, Fleming JE, Boehm CA, et al. Aspiration of osteoprogenitor cells for augmenting spinal fusion: comparison of progenitor cell concentrations from the vertebral body and iliac crest. J Bone Joint Surg Am 2005;87(12):2655–61.

23. Hyer CF, Berlet GC, Bussewitz BW, et al. Quantitative assessment of the yield of osteoblastic connective tissue progenitors in bone marrow aspirate from the iliac crest, tibia, and calcaneus. J Bone Joint Surg Am 2013;95(14):1312–6.

24. Pierini M, Di Bella C, Dozza B, et al. The posterior iliac crest outperforms the anterior iliac crest when obtaining mesenchymal stem cells from bone marrow. J Bone Joint Surg Am 2013;95(12):1101–7.

25. Marx RE, Tursun R. A qualitative and quantitative analysis of autologous human multipotent adult stem cells derived from three anatomic areas by marrow aspiration: tibia, anterior ilium, and posterior ilium. Int J Oral Maxillofac Implants 2013;28(5):e290–4.

26. Hernigou P, Homma Y, Flouzat Lachaniette CH, et al. Benefits of small volume and small syringe for bone marrow aspirations of mesenchymal stem cells. Int Orthop 2013;37(11):2279–87.

Large BM Intra-Articular Allograft

Joan R. Williams, MD[a],*, Michael E. Brage, MD[b]

KEYWORDS

• Allograft • Arthroplasty • Posttraumatic ankle arthritis

KEY POINTS

• Intra-articular allograft is an alternative treatment of posttraumatic ankle arthritis.
• Allografts should be implanted as close to the time of procurement as possible to enhance the success of the procedure.
• Improper graft cuts or size mismatch have an increased risk of graft failure.
• Failure of allograft can be salvaged with a revision arthrodesis.

INTRODUCTION: NATURE OF THE PROBLEM

Severe posttraumatic tibiotalar arthritis can be a challenge to treat in young patients. After these patients fail to respond to conservative treatment options, such as bracing, physical therapy, corticosteroid injections, and activity modifications, surgical treatment options typically include ankle arthrodesis or total ankle arthroplasty.[1–8]

Ankle arthrodesis has been shown to alleviate pain in the arthritic ankle. However, loss of range of motion, functional limitation, and secondary progressive arthritis in the hindfoot and midfoot have been found in long-term follow-up studies on patients with isolated ankle arthrodesis.[2]

Current total ankle prosthetic designs are a promising alternative to arthrodesis, but patients' age has an adverse affect on the risk of failure and reoperation rate.[8–10] Osteochondral shell allografting, in which the tibial plafond and talar dome are replaced with a donor ankle matched for size, affords relief of pain, congruent articular surfaces, maintenance of bone stock, and preservation of surrounding joints. Recent improvements in surgical techniques and experience with allografts have improved short-term outcomes with this technique.[11–13]

The authors have nothing to disclose.
[a] UCLA Department of Orthopaedic Surgery, 1250 16th Street, Suite 3142, Santa Monica, CA 90404, USA; [b] Department of Orthopaedic Surgery, University of Washington, Seattle, WA, USA
* Corresponding author.
E-mail address: joanryanwilliams@gmail.com

INDICATIONS/CONTRAINDICATIONS

This procedure is typically used in patients with posttraumatic ankle arthritis who wish to retain joint motion but are too young to undergo total ankle arthroplasty. Relative contraindications included inflammatory arthritis, the presence of active infection, or deformity or instability of the ankle that is not passively correctable. Additionally, an allograft that is size matched to patients needs to be obtained before this surgery.

SURGICAL TECHNIQUE/PROCEDURE
Preoperative Planning

All patients should undergo a thorough history and physical examination. Standard weight-bearing radiographs of the ankle (anteroposterior [AP], mortise, lateral) should be obtained and reviewed. From these images a size-matched osteochondral allograft needs to be obtained from a regional tissue bank.

PREP AND PATIENT POSITIONING

Patients are placed supine on a radiolucent table. A thigh tourniquet may be used if desired.

SURGICAL APPROACH

A standard anterior approach to the ankle is used. This approach uses the interval between the tibialis anterior and extensor halluces longus tendons. Care should be taken to protect the superficial peroneal nerve during the superficial dissection. The deep neurovascular bundle is retracted laterally, and the ankle joint is exposed by an anterior capsulotomy.

Surgical Procedure

1. Through the anterior approach, excise synovitis and remove osteophytes using rongeurs and osteotomes. Next, apply an external fixator to distract the joint symmetrically about 1 cm.
2. Examine the arthritic ankle to determine whether a hemiarthroplasty or total arthroplasty is needed to fix the osteochondral defect.
3. Determine the ideal Agility (DePuy, Warsaw, IN) cutting block by templating the preoperative ankle radiographs. Pin the corresponding Agility ankle arthroplasty cutting block into place over the anterior ankle (**Fig. 1**). Confirm the placement and size with intraoperative fluoroscopy.
4. Using a blunt reciprocating saw, resect the tibial plafond and talar dome to a thickness of about 7 to 10 mm.
5. Remove an articular portion of the medial malleolus (about 3–4 mm) as well with care to protect the posteromedial neurovascular bundle.
6. Prepare the allograft. The Agility ankle cutting block for the tibial cut of the donor graft is one size larger than the block used on the recipient tibia. Pin the cutting block onto the graft and confirm the position by using fluoroscopy, and then make the cut with an oscillating saw (**Fig. 2**).
7. Cut the talus allograft free hand using an oscillating saw. The cut is made at the interface between the anterior neck and cartilage. The authors routinely lavage both the tibial and talar grafts to remove immunogenic marrow elements (**Fig. 3**).

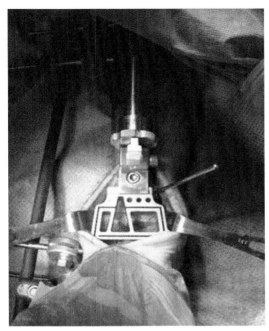

Fig. 1. Exposure of the ankle joint with the medially based external fixator and Agility cutting jig in place.

8. With the ankle in plantar flexion, seat the grafts into the recipient mortise. Remove the external fixator and take the ankle through a range of motion to confirm graft and ankle stability.
9. Imaging in the AP, mortise, and lateral planes confirms that the grafts have satisfactory apposition to the host bone and that the anatomy of the tibiotalar joint has been restored.

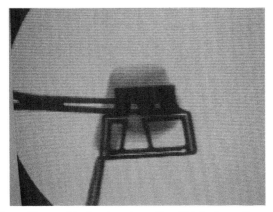

Fig. 2. The Agility cutting guide is placed on the tibial allograft and confirmed with fluoroscopy.

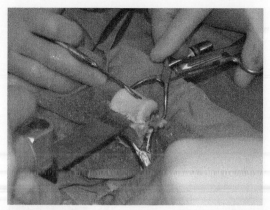

Fig. 3. The talar allograft is cut by hand using an oscillating saw at the interface between the anterior neck and the cartilage.

10. Place 2 parallel 3.0-mm cannulated screws into the tibia from the anterior portion of the tibial graft into the recipient tibia while aiming superiorly and posteriorly.
11. Place 2 fixation screws on the anterior portion of the talar graft into the native talus through the most anterior portion of the articular cartilage. Countersink these screws into subchondral bone (**Fig. 4**).
12. Perform copious irrigation and routine wound closure, and place patients in a bulky cotton splint.

COMPLICATIONS AND MANAGEMENT

The main complications seen with this procedure are intraoperative fracture, graft collapse, poor graft fixation, nonunion, and need for additional debridement postoperatively. If an intraoperative fracture of the malleoli occurs, it should be fixed at that time. Problems with graft fixation or nonunion can be treated in a secondary procedure with either revision allograft or arthrodesis depending on the reason for failure and patients' desires (**Fig. 5**).

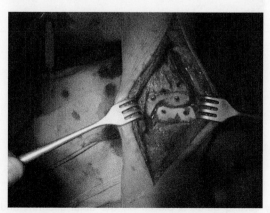

Fig. 4. The allograft is in place and is held with countersunk 3.0-mm cannulated screws.

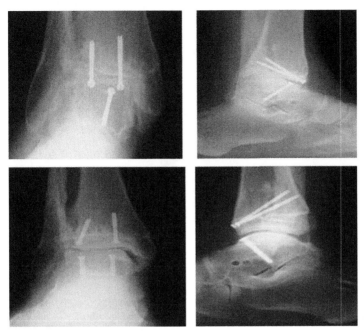

Fig. 5. The top row shows an AP and lateral radiograph of a patient 2 years postoperatively from the original allograft in which the joint space has again narrowed. The patient was revised to a second allograft, which is shown in the bottom row.

POSTOPERATIVE CARE

Perioperative antibiotics and pain control are at the surgeon's discretion. Patients are placed in a bulky cotton splint with the ankle in neutral to slight dorsiflexion postoperatively. Range-of-motion exercises are started when the wound has healed, typically at postoperative day 10. The authors routinely keep the operated extremity at touchdown weight bearing for 3 months and then progress to weight bearing as tolerated as long as there are satisfactory radiographs that suggest progression toward graft incorporation.

OUTCOMES

Promising case series have reported on total ankle osteochondral shell allograft replacement of the tibiotalar joint as a viable alternative for posttraumatic ankle arthritis in young patients.[11–13] The largest case series to date reports 6 out of 11 successful grafting procedures at a minimum follow-up of 24 months. Of the other 5 patients, 3 had revision allografting and one was revised to total ankle arthroplasty. The last patient did not have any further surgery.[12] **Fig. 6** shows preoperative and 6-year postoperative radiographs of a patient who successfully underwent bulk allograft transplant for posttraumatic ankle arthritis.

Jeng and Myerson reported that 14 of 29 fresh osteochondral shell allograft transplants had been revised to a repeat ankle transplant/arthrodesis. Six of the remaining 15 allografts were radiographic failures with progressive loss of joint space but did not require revision surgery. The remaining 9 allografts (31%) were deemed a success. The investigators concluded that patients with a lower body mass index, less angular

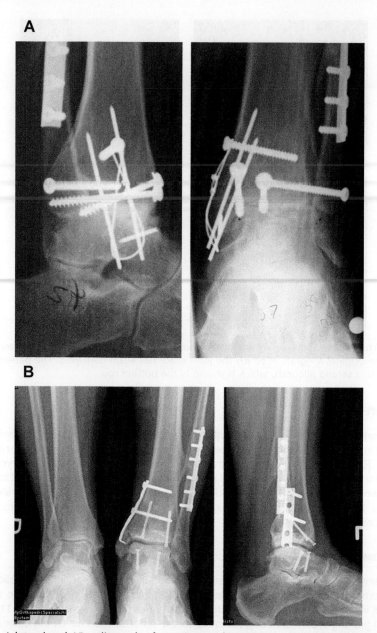

Fig. 6. A lateral and AP radiograph of a patient with posttraumatic ankle arthritis after a pilon fracture (*A*). An AP and lateral radiograph of a patient who underwent bulk allograft transplant at 6 years postoperatively (*B*).

deformity, and who refused arthrodesis did better. These investigators did not use an external fixator during the procedure and did not use a cutting block one size bigger for the allograft as suggested in this article. Therefore, their grafts may have been small/thin. Grafts should be at least 7 mm thick to prevent collapse.[14]

Gross and colleagues[4] reported on 9 patients treated with large fresh allografts of the talus to treat osteochondral lesions (OCD) lesions. Of the 9 patients, 6 had successful procedures and remained in situ with a mean survival of 11 years. Three patients had fragmentation and collapse of the grafts and were converted to arthrodeses.

Giannini and colleagues[15] reported on 32 patients treated with bipolar allografts via a lateral transmalleolar approach. Of the 32 patients, 9 required revision at the time of the latest follow-up of 31 months. They also examined cartilage samples from 7 of the patients at 1 year of follow-up finding hyalinelike histology with normal collagen; however, it was more disorganized than native cartilage and had less proteoglycan content. They also delayed weight bearing for 6 months, which they think may have increased their success rate.[15]

Neri and colleagues[16–18] examined the genotypic and phenotypic characterizations of transplanted osteochondral allograft in 17 patients and found a prevalence of host DNA in retrieved allografts suggesting incorporation.[12]

Multiple studies have listed graft-host size mismatch, excessively thin cuts, elevated body mass index, and degree of preoperative deformity as risk factors for graft failure. They have also discussed that decreased time between harvesting of the allograft and implantation may increase success.[13,14,19–21]

SUMMARY

Osteochondral shell allograft is a treatment option for posttraumatic ankle arthritis in young patients who wish to preserve joint motion and are not candidates for total ankle arthroplasty with metal prostheses. Overall, this technique proves improved ankle function in most patients. In situations whereby the allograft fails, arthrodesis remains an option.

REFERENCES

1. Abidi NA, Gruen GS, Conti SF. Ankle arthrodesis: indications and techniques. J Am Acad Orthop Surg 2000;8:200–9.
2. Coester LM, Saltzman CL, Leupold J, et al. Long-term results following ankle arthrodesis for post-traumatic arthritis. J Bone Joint Surg Am 2001;83-A:219–28.
3. Coughlin MJ, Mann RA. Surgery of the foot and ankle. St Louis (MO): Mosby; 1999.
4. Gross AE, Agnidis Z, Hutchison CR. Osteochondral defects of the talus treated with fresh osteochondral allograft transplantation. Foot Ankle Int 2001;22(5): 385–91.
5. Haddad SL, Coetzee JC, Estok R, et al. Intermediate and long-term outcomes of total ankle arthroplasty and ankle arthrodesis a systematic review of the literature. J Bone Joint Surg Am 2007;89:1899–905.
6. Hansen ST. Functional reconstruction of the foot and ankle. Philadelphia: Lippincott Williams & Wilkins; 2000.
7. Mann RA, Rongstad KM. Arthrodesis of the ankle: a critical analysis. Foot Ankle Int 1998;19:3–9.
8. Spirt AA, Assal M, Hansen ST. Complications and failure after total ankle arthroplasty. J Bone Joint Surg Am 2004;86-A:1172–8.
9. Kitaoka HB, Patzer GL, Ilstrup DM, et al. Survivorship analysis of the Mayo total ankle arthroplasty. J Bone Joint Surg Am 1994;76-A:974–9.
10. SooHoo NF, Zingmond DS, Ko CY. Comparison of reoperation rates following ankle arthrodesis and total ankle arthrplasty. J Bone Joint Surg Am 2007;89: 2143–9.

11. Kim CW, Jamali A, Tontz W, et al. Treatment of post-traumatic ankle arthrosis with bipolar tibiotalar osteochondral shell allografts. Foot Ankle Int 2002;23:1091–102.

12. Meehan R, McFarlin S, Bugbee W, et al. Fresh ankle osteochondral allograft transplantation for tibiotalar joint arthritis. Foot Ankle Int 2005;26:793–802.

13. Tontz W, Bugbee W, Brage ME. Use of allografts in the management of ankle arthritis. Foot Ankle Clin 2003;8:361–73.

14. Jeng CL, Myerson MS. Fresh osteochondral total ankle allograft transplantation for the treatment of ankle arthritis. Foot Ankle Clin 2008;13:539–47.

15. Giannini S, Buda R, Grigolo B, et al. Bipolar fresh osteochondral allograft of the ankle. Foot Ankle Int 2010;31(1):38–46.

16. Neri S, Vannini F, Desando G, et al. Ankle bipolar fresh osteochondral allograft survivorship and integration: transplanted tissue genetic typing and phenotypic characteristics. J Bone Joint Surg Am 2013;95:1852–60.

17. Reider B. The orthopaedic physical exam. Philadelphia: Elsevier; 2005.

18. Richardson EG. Orthopaedic knowledge update: foot and ankle 3. Rosemont (IL): American Academy of Orthopaedic Surgeons; 2004.

19. Strauss EJ, Sershon R, Barker JU, et al. The basic science and clinical applications of osteochondral allografts. Bull NYU Hosp Jt Dis 2012;70(4):217–23.

20. Thomas RH, Daniels TR. Current concepts review ankle arthritis. J Bone Joint Surg Am 2003;85-A:923–36.

21. Winters BS, Raikin SM. The use of allograft in joint preserving surgery for ankle osteochondral lesions and osteoarthritis. Foot Ankle Clin 2013;18:529–42.

Efficacy of a Cellular Allogeneic Bone Graft in Foot and Ankle Arthrodesis Procedures

 CrossMark

Travis J. Dekker, MD, Peter White, MD, Samuel B. Adams, MD*

KEYWORDS

- Map3 • Allograft • Arthrodesis • MAPCs • Foot • Ankle • Nonunion • Stem cell

KEY POINTS

- The use of a cellular allogeneic bone graft is safe and effective in foot and ankle arthrodesis patients with risk factors known to cause nonunion.
- Map3 provided an overall fusion rate of 83% in a mostly high-risk population for nonunion.
- The use of this cellular allogeneic bone graft nullified the risk of nonunion for patients with infection, previous nonunion, avascular necrosis, and positive smoking status.
- Diabetes was the only independent risk factor for arthrodesis nonunion, despite the use of Map3 in this patient population.
- Patients with diabetes must be counseled about the risk of nonunion despite the use of supplemental biological therapy for arthrodesis procedures.

INTRODUCTION

Arthrodesis remains the gold standard treatment of end-stage arthritis of the foot and ankle. However, fusion is not guaranteed. Many patients have comorbidities that portend to an increase risk of nonunion, including smoking, diabetes, and avascular necrosis, among others. In various ways, all of these comorbidities compromise vascularity and in turn the delivery of nutrients and host reparative cells to the arthrodesis site. Attempting arthrodesis in these high-risk patients has led to nonunion rates as high as 40%, which can lead to persistent pain and debilitation.[1–4]

In 1965, Urist[5] demonstrated the ability of autologous graft to differentiate and form bone due to bone morphogenetic proteins demonstrating the osteoinductive properties of autograft. Today, autograft is considered the gold standard bone graft as it

Dr. Adams is a paid consultant for rti surgical.
Department of Orthopaedic Surgery, Duke University Medical Center, Erwin Road, Durham, NC 27710, USA
* Corresponding author. Duke University Medical Center, 4709 Creekstone Drive, Durham, NC 27703.
E-mail address: Samuel.adams@duke.edu

Foot Ankle Clin N Am 21 (2016) 855–861
http://dx.doi.org/10.1016/j.fcl.2016.07.008
1083-7515/16/© 2016 Elsevier Inc. All rights reserved.

foot.theclinics.com

attempts to stimulate local biology at nonunion sites as it provides the essential elements of bone formation: osteoconduction, osteoinduction, and osteogenicity.[6] To increase the union rate, autologous bone graft is used to enhance bone healing at primary arthrodesis and revision nonunion sites. Autologous bone graft is often supplemented even in primary surgical procedures in patients that are at high risk of nonunion with the comorbidities outlined earlier or the presence of a bone void at the arthrodesis site.

However, the incidence of complications and postoperative morbidity after autograft bone harvest has been reported to be as high as 23%.[7] These complications include donor-site pain, infection, fracture, seroma, wound complications, sensory loss, and scarring.[8] In addition, autograft collection is not a viable option for every patient, with limitations associated with the available supply of graft material or variability in the quantity and quality of osteoprogenitor cells present in patients with advanced age or medical comorbidities. Therefore, many attempts have been made to produce allogeneic bone graft supplements with the elements essential for increased bone growth and the avoidance of morbidity of autologous bone graft harvesting.

Allogeneic bone grafts are a viable alternative to avoid the possible complications associated with the collection of autograft bone. This study reports on the use of Map3 (RTI, Alachua, Florida) cellular allogeneic bone graft. The allograft contains cortical cancellous bone chips that serve as an osteoconductive scaffold, demineralized bone matrix (DBM) with verified osteoinductive potential, and viable multipotent adult progenitor-class (MAPC) cells capable of osteogenesis and the production of angiogenic signals to support the bone healing process.

The purpose of this study was to review of use of Map3 cellular allogeneic bone graft in foot and ankle arthrodesis surgeries in patients with risk factors that have been previously shown to increase the rate of nonunion. This study evaluates the clinical effectiveness of Map3 cellular allogeneic bone graft and reports resulting complications in this patient cohort.

METHODS

An Institutional Review Board–approved retrospective chart review was performed at a single academic institution. Patients in this case series underwent foot or ankle arthrodesis that required use of Map3 cellular allogeneic bone graft to fill a bony defect at the time of arthrodesis surgery. In all cases, Map3 was placed in the bony defect between the two intended healing surfaces (prepared joint surfaces). A foot and ankle fellowship-trained orthopedic surgeon with extensive experience in complex ankle and hindfoot reconstruction procedures performed all surgeries.

Clinical records were obtained to determine patient demographics, comorbidities, fixation methods, use of biological adjuvants at the time of surgery, union outcome, and complications. The authors' primary objective was to determine the effectiveness of achieving radiographic union in the setting of patients at risk for nonunion. Fusion was defined by consensus between 2 foot and ankle fellowship-trained investigators after assessing the radiographs and computed tomography (CT) scans when available. Successful radiographic fusion required the presence of bridging bone, no radiographic signs of nonunion, maintenance of fixation across the surgical site as previously defined,[9] and resolution of preoperative symptoms. CT scans were obtained at the treating surgeon's discretion.

Student t-tests were used to assess fusion rates comparing all comorbidities in a univariate analysis. A 2-by-2 contingency table and Fisher exact test of independence were used to compare fusion rates using Map3 alone versus Map3 with additional adjuvants. Statistical analyses were performed on JMP version 12 (SAS, Cary, NC). Statistical significance was set at $P<.05$.

RESULTS

This study consisted of 23 patients, with a mean age at surgery of 51.5 years (range, 19–73 years) and a mean follow-up of 15 months (range, 12–24 months). **Table 1** details the arthrodesis sites. The overall fusion rate in this cohort was 82.6% (19 of 23), with one (4.7%) reported complication of a surgical site infection requiring irrigation and debridement.

Most patients (17 of 23, 74%) had at least one comorbidity known to place them at risk for nonunion.[1–3] Overall fusion rates for each individual risk factor can be seen in **Table 2**. In univariate analysis, diabetes was the only independent risk factor ($P<.001$) for recurrent nonunion, whereas all other independent risk factors (smoking, avascular necrosis [AVN], nonunion, infection) did not portend an increased risk of nonunion in this patient cohort with use of Map3 (**Table 3**). Furthermore, the number of comorbidities did not independently increase the risk of nonunion. Lastly, no significant difference existed in fusion rate when Map3 was used alone or in combination with another bone graft or orthobiologic (femoral head allograft, allograft cancellous chips, concentrated bone marrow aspirate, bone morphogenic protein), indicating lack of need to use additional biologics with Map3.

DISCUSSION

This case series demonstrated successful fusion in complicated arthrodesis procedures of the foot and ankle and provided initial data to support the use of a cellular allogeneic bone graft substitute as a potential alternative to iliac crest autograft.

Arthrodesis is a common surgical procedure that can reduce pain and improve function in patients with arthritis and deformities of the foot and ankle. The goal of arthrodesis is to create ossification (fusion) between 2 bones. In ankle and hindfoot fusions, nonunion continues to be a major concern because it occurs in approximately 10% of these procedures. However, the nonunion rate increases to 16% to 41% in patients with a history of smoking, diabetes, and AVN, all of which limit achieving well-vascularized bony surfaces for fusion to take place.[2,3] The lack of vascularity at the site creates an additional hurdle on the rate of healing as the presence of blood vessels is key to allow for the necessary nutrients and host cells to migrate to the site of repair and begin the healing response.

To increase the union rate, autologous bone graft has been used to enhance bone healing at primary arthrodesis and revision nonunion sites. This is especially true in

Table 1
Arthrodesis sites and nonunion rate

Joint	N = 23	Number of Nonunions
Ankle	6	1
Subtalar	1	0
Tibiotalocalcaneal	10	1
Midfoot	3	2
First metatarsophalangeal	2	0
Fibula nonunion	1	0

Table 2
Fusion rate for each risk factor

Risk Factor	N	Overall % of Cohort	Number Fused	% Fused
Smoking	7	30	6	86
Diabetes	4	17	1	25
Avascular necrosis	4	17	3	75
Previous nonunion	7	30	5	71
Previous infection	5	22	4	80

cases whereby patients exhibit bony defects or the risk factors outlined earlier. Autograft is considered by some as the gold standard bone graft because it can provide the essential elements of bone formation: osteoconduction, osteoinduction, and osteogenicity.[6] However, the incidence of complications and postoperative morbidity after autograft bone harvest has been reported to be as high as 23%.[7] These complications include donor-site pain, infection, fracture, seroma, wound complications, sensory loss, and scarring.[8] In addition, autograft collection is not a viable alternative for every patient, as there might be limitations associated with the available supply of graft material or variability in the quantity and quality of osteoprogenitor cells present in patients with advanced age or medical comorbidities.

Allogeneic bone grafts are a viable alternative to avoid the possible complications associated with the collection of autograft material. An ideal bone graft substitute, to fill voids or promote healing, provides an osteoconductive matrix combined with osteoinductive signals and viable cells with osteogenic potential. Map3 is a human cellular allogeneic bone graft that provides the components essential to optimal fracture healing. The implant contains cortical cancellous bone chips that serve as an osteoconductive scaffold, DBM with verified osteoinductive potential, and viable MAPCs with osteogenic and angiogenic signals to support the bone healing process.

Data on the use of cellular allogeneic bone graft in foot and ankle surgery are limited. Jones and colleagues[9] reported on 76 patients with a 1-year follow-up in a prospective multicenter trial on the use of a cellular allogeneic bone matrix for foot and ankle arthrodesis procedures. They reported a 71.1% fusion rate at 12 months for this

Table 3
Risk factor subgroup analysis

	Risk Factor	%	P Value
Smoking	Smoker fusion rate	86	.4
	Nonsmoker fusion rate	81	
Diabetes	Diabetes fusion rate	25	<.001
	Nondiabetic fusion rate	95	
AVN	AVN fusion rate	75	.33
	No AVN fusion rate	84	
Previous nonunion	Previous nonunion fusion rate	71	.19
	No previous nonunion fusion rate	88	
Previous infection	Previous infection fusion rate	80	.43
	No previous infection fusion rate	83	

patient population and concluded that this fusion rate was comparable with what was reported in the literature when autograft was used.

With regard to risk factors for nonunion, smoking decreases the oxygen saturation at the cellular level of the tissue mediated by the vasoconstrictive and platelet-aggregating effects of nicotine, the inhibition of oxidative metabolism due to hydrogen cyanide, and, lastly, the hypoxemic effects of carbon dioxide.[10,11] Furthermore, smoking has been shown in both animal and human models to increase the risk of nonunion and also prolong or delay union if it fusion is eventually achieved.[3,12–15] Despite the known increase to go onto nonunion, the use of Map3 in smoking patients made the fusion rates near equivalent with 85.7% of smokers versus 81.3% in nonsmokers in this cohort with no significant difference between the groups.

AVN by definition lacks the necessary vascularity to delivery both oxygen and essential nutrients necessary for bone healing. Animal models have demonstrated that without vascular endothelial growth factor, both intramembranous and endochondral pathways of osteogenesis are inhibited. Clinical findings confirm this with Easley and colleagues[3] reporting a decreased subtalar fusion rate of 22% in patients with AVN. One element of the Map3 bone graft is the MAPCs. Animal studies have shown that MAPC cells can generate and sustain vascular cells and tissue.[16] The authors' findings demonstrate with the use of Map3, patients with AVN have comparable fusion rates with those who do not.

Although to the authors' knowledge no literature reports fusion rates after infection in foot and ankle fusions, the trauma literature clearly associates increased rates of nonunion and delayed healing in the setting of infection.[17,18] Infection delays healing on the cellular level altering cell function and viability.[19] Interestingly, the authors' data demonstrate near-equivalent fusion rates despite prior history of same surgical site infection (80% vs 83%, $P = .43$). Furthermore, the use of Map3 did not place patients at higher risk of persistent infection, as no patient with a history of prior infection of the involved bones to be fused required any further operative intervention for infection.

Diabetes impairs bone healing and fusion through a variety of mechanisms. Al-Aql and colleagues[20] demonstrated that diabetes leads to delayed ossification and impairment of collagen synthesis, whereas more recently McCabe[21] and Shimoaka and colleagues[22] have shown hyperglycemia paired with hypoinsulinemia directly impairs bone generation. Furthermore, O'Connor and colleagues[4] recently demonstrated clinical evidence that diabetic patients have an increased risk of nonunion in attempts at revision arthrodesis. Other larger cohorts have demonstrated similar results with nonunion rates nearly 10% higher compared with nondiabetic patients.[19] The authors' findings corroborate these conclusions with a statistically significant difference in diabetic patients regardless of the addition of Map3 as an adjuvant. Challenging patients with diabetes continues to be a significant risk factor for persistent nonunion and pain even 1 year out from surgery. When attempting arthrodesis in diabetic patients, extensive counseling should be administered before surgery about risks of nonunion and need for further and more extensive operations.

Despite these promising preliminary results, the investigative use of Map3 for fusion requires further research and evaluation. The data derived from this small cohort offer an alternative to other graft sources with reproducible and significant results. The data obtained are both retrospective and from a small cohort with limited follow-up, which can ultimately lead to intrinsic bias in this study. The continued use in this unique population subset requires longer follow-up and larger sample sizes to be obtained prospectively.

SUMMARY

Map3 is a novel cellular allogeneic bone graft substitute with all elements of an ideal bone graft with allograft bone chips acting as an osteoconductive scaffold, demineralized bone matrix providing osteoinduction, MAPC cells with osteogenic, and angiogenic properties. The use of Map3 in arthrodeses can help minimize the risk of nonunion in smokers, revision arthrodesis cases, AVN, and infection. Analysis with larger samples and longer follow-up are future areas of this orthobiologic intervention that can further expand indications, efficacy, and reliability.

REFERENCES

1. DiGiovanni CW, Lin SS, Baumhauer JF, et al. Recombinant human platelet-derived growth factor-BB and beta-tricalcium phosphate (rhPDGF-BB/beta-TCP): an alternative to autogenous bone graft. J Bone Joint Surg Am 2013; 95(13):1184–92.
2. Frey C, Halikus NM, Vu-Rose T, et al. A review of ankle arthrodesis: predisposing factors to nonunion. Foot Ankle Int 1994;15(11):581–4.
3. Easley ME, Trnka HJ, Schon LC, et al. Isolated subtalar arthrodesis. J Bone Joint Surg Am 2000;82(5):613–24.
4. O'Connor KM, Johnson JE, McCormick JJ, et al. Clinical and operative factors related to successful revision arthrodesis in the foot and ankle. Foot Ankle Int 2016;37(8):809–15.
5. Urist MR. Bone: formation by autoinduction. Science 1965;150(3698):893–9.
6. Yaszemski MJ, Payne RG, Hayes WC, et al. Evolution of bone transplantation: molecular, cellular and tissue strategies to engineer human bone. Biomaterials 1996;17(2):175–85.
7. Ahlmann E, Patzakis M, Roidis N, et al. Comparison of anterior and posterior iliac crest bone grafts in terms of harvest-site morbidity and functional outcomes. J Bone Joint Surg Am 2002;84-A(5):716–20.
8. DiGiovanni CW, Petricek JM. The evolution of rhPDGF-BB in musculoskeletal repair and its role in foot and ankle fusion surgery. Foot Ankle Clin 2010;15(4): 621–40.
9. Jones CP, Loveland J, Atkinson BL, et al. Prospective, multicenter evaluation of allogeneic bone matrix containing viable osteogenic cells in foot and/or ankle arthrodesis. Foot Ankle Int 2015;36(10):1129–37.
10. Lawrence WT, Murphy RC, Robson MC, et al. The detrimental effect of cigarette smoking on flap survival: an experimental study in the rat. Br J Plast Surg 1984; 37(2):216–9.
11. Campanile G, Hautmann G, Lotti T. Cigarette smoking, wound healing, and facelift. Clin Dermatol 1998;16(5):575–8.
12. Murray IR, Foster CJ, Eros A, et al. Risk factors for nonunion after nonoperative treatment of displaced midshaft fractures of the clavicle. J Bone Joint Surg Am 2013;95(13):1153–8.
13. Chahal J, Stephen DJ, Bulmer B, et al. Factors associated with outcome after subtalar arthrodesis. J Orthop Trauma 2006;20(8):555–61.
14. Adams CI, Keating JF, Court-Brown CM. Cigarette smoking and open tibial fractures. Injury 2001;32(1):61–5.
15. Krannitz KW, Fong HW, Fallat LM, et al. The effect of cigarette smoking on radiographic bone healing after elective foot surgery. J Foot Ankle Surg 2009;48(5): 525–7.

16. Aranguren XL, McCue JD, Hendrickx B, et al. Multipotent adult progenitor cells sustain function of ischemic limbs in mice. J Clin Invest 2008;118(2):505–14.

17. Malik MH, Harwood P, Diggle P, et al. Factors affecting rates of infection and nonunion in intramedullary nailing. J Bone Joint Surg Br 2004;86(4):556–60.

18. Baldwin KD, Babatunde OM, Russell Huffman G, et al. Open fractures of the tibia in the pediatric population: a systematic review. J Child Orthop 2009;3(3): 199–208.

19. Perlman MH, Thordarson DB. Ankle fusion in a high risk population: an assessment of nonunion risk factors. Foot Ankle Int 1999;20(8):491–6.

20. Ai-Aql ZS, Alagl AS, Graves DT, et al. Molecular mechanisms controlling bone formation during fracture healing and distraction osteogenesis. J Dent Res 2008; 87(2):107–18.

21. McCabe LR. Understanding the pathology and mechanisms of type I diabetic bone loss. J Cell Biochem 2007;102(6):1343–57.

22. Shimoaka T, Kamekura S, Chikuda H, et al. Impairment of bone healing by insulin receptor substrate-1 deficiency. J Biol Chem 2004;279(15):15314–22.

The Use of Allostem in Subtalar Fusions

J. Chris Coetzee, MD[a],*, Mark S. Myerson, MD[b], John G. Anderson, MD[c]

KEYWORDS

- Subtalar fusions • Augmentation • Mesenchymal stem cells

KEY POINTS

- No orthobiologic adjuvant will substitute for poor surgical technique.
- Diligent joint preparation is critical to success of any arthrodesis.
- Optimal joint preparation is important, but there is a risk of vascular compromise to the bone if all 3 facets of the subtalar joint are aggressively prepared, because it requires stripping of the soft tissues in the sinus tarsi, which may potentially compromise local vascularity.
- Fusing the posterior facet alone is often sufficient in cases without fixed varus or valgus deformity.
- Subtalar arthrodesis takes a long time to mature, and rehabilitation should be planned accordingly with appropriate immobilization and restricted bearing of weight.

INTRODUCTION: NATURE OF THE PROBLEM

The rate of union following subtalar arthrodesis is not predictable, albeit poor in some studies, with the reported nonunion rate varying from 5% to 45%. In the largest study in the literature, by Easley and coworkers,[1] the union rate was 84% (154 of 184) in the group as a whole, with 86% (134 of 156) overall after primary arthrodesis, and 71% (20 of 28) in the group of patients who had undergone a previous attempted arthrodesis with failure.

Several of the other articles in this issue deal with other options to try to increase arthrodesis rates in foot and ankle arthrodesis. Bear in mind, however, that in the most extensive prospective randomized study to date, one of the conclusions was that "the primary effectiveness end point was met: twenty-four-week arthrodesis rates for rhPDGF-BB/b-TCP as assessed by means of CT were found to be non-inferior (equivalent) to those for autograft."[2] In the latter study, other than donor site morbidity

The study was sponsored by AlloSource, Centennial, CO.

[a] Twin Cities Orthopedics, 4010 West 65th Street, Edina, MN 55435, USA; [b] The Foot and Ankle Association Inc., Institute for Foot and Ankle Recon at Mercy, 301 Saint Paul Place, Baltimore, MD 21202, USA; [c] Orthopaedic Associates of Michigan, 230 Michigan Northeast, Suite 300, Grand Rapids, MI 4950, USA
* Corresponding author.
E-mail address: jcc@tcomn.com

where the rhPDGF-BB/b-TCP could have a higher score, as a pure substitute, it appears to be equivalent, and not better than autograft.

In the ongoing search for an alternative that is equal or better than autologous graft, the authors explored the option of using human mesenchymal stem cells (MSC). Even though embryonic stem cells have massive potential, many ethical and political issues occur with their use, and the goal therefore has been to find MSCs in adult tissue that are comparable in activity and use.

Musina and coworkers[3] looked at the quality of stem cells obtained from different human tissues and investigated bone marrow (iliac crest), adipose tissue, placenta, thymus, and skin, where the stem cells were isolated and cultured under identical conditions.

Their conclusion included the following[3]:

- MSC were found in all the tissue types.
- Subcutaneous adipose tissue had a much higher MSC count than bone marrow in the same donors.
- The cells from different sources had similar morphologic characteristics and gene expression.
- Adipose tissue and thymus MSCs proliferated the quickest, whereas placenta proliferated the slowest.
- The older the donor, the lower the MSC count and the slower the proliferation.

Zuk and coworkers[4] also looked at human adipose tissue as a source of MSCs.[4] They did an exhaustive study looking at multiple variables and concluded that adult human adipose–derived MSCs have multilineage potential and can undergo the following:

- Differentiation into adipose tissue
- Osteogenic differentiation
- Chondrogenic differentiation
- Myogenic differentiation
- Neurogenic differentiation

With these and other studies that confirmed that adipose-derived MSCs could be a relatively simple augment to arthrodesis, the authors decided to embark on a prospective randomized multicenter study comparing subtalar arthrodesis with either autologous bone graft or Allostem (AllosSource, Centennial, CO, USA).

Allostem is partially demineralized allograft bone combined with adipose-derived MSCs. The partially demineralized allograft bone is osteoconductive and osteoinductive, whereas the MSCs is osteogenic and may contribute to new bone formation.

Allostem comes in different configurations, and the flat strips were chosen for the study (**Fig. 1**).

STUDY DESIGN

Institutional review board (IRB) approval was obtained from 4 different sites to embark on a prospective randomized noninferiority study to compare Allostem with autologous bone graft for subtalar arthrodesis.

INDICATIONS/CONTRAINDICATIONS

The authors attempted to make the inclusion and exclusion criteria as simple and narrow as possible to prevent multiple variables that could skew the results. The criteria are outlined in **Box 1**.

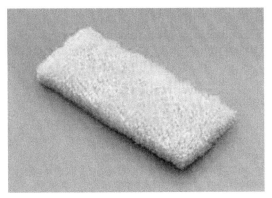

Fig. 1. Allostem strips were used for the study. It is partially demineralized allograft bone combined with adipose-derived MSCs.

SURGICAL TECHNIQUE/PROCEDURE
Preoperative Planning

IRB approval was obtained for the study for all the research sites. When patients were enrolled, weight-bearing radiographs were done preoperatively as well as completion of the American Orthopedic Foot and Ankle Society (AOFAS) Ankle-Hindfoot Scale, Foot Function Index-long form (FFI-R), Short Form-12 (SF-12), Visual Analog Pain Scale (VAS), and a clinical questionnaire.

These items were completed at the same intervals as the radiographs at weeks 6 and 12, 3 months, 6 months, and 1 year.

PREPARATION AND PATIENT POSITIONING

The usual surgical approach was used for a subtalar arthrodesis with the patient supine with a bump under the ipsilateral buttock. A thigh tourniquet was used, and the leg sterilely prepared and draped to include exposure of the knee.

Box 1
A description of both inclusion and exclusion criteria

Inclusion criteria

Age 18–80

Anyone that needs an isolated ST arthrodesis (posttraumatic, rheumatoid, primary degenerative joint disease)

Willing and able to comply with the clinical trial protocol

Exclusion criteria

Younger than 18, older than 80

Peripheral neuropathy or peripheral vascular insufficiency

Severely deformed hindfoot that would require major osteotomies or multijoint arthrodesis

Infection or history of infection

Received treatment within the past 12 months that may interfere with bone metabolism (bisphosphonates, therapeutic doses of vitamin D, calcitonin)

SURGICAL APPROACH

A standard sinus tarsi incision was used to expose the subtalar joint. The authors prefer a longitudinal incision from the tip of the fibula to the anterior process of the calcaneus.

SURGICAL PROCEDURE

The posterior and middle facets were exposed and denuded of cartilage. The opposing surfaces were also feathered with a small osteotome and/or a burr or drill to expose subchondral bone.

In group A, autologous graft was harvested from either the medial distal tibia or the proximal tibia and placed in the posterior facet and sinus tarsi.

In group B, 1 strip of Allostem was placed in a divot in the posterior facet, and 1 strip was placed in the sinus tarsi.

Stable internal fixation with one or two 6.5- or 7.0-mm partial threaded screws were then used to provide initial stability and compression at the arthrodesis site.

COMPLICATIONS AND MANAGEMENT

There were no complications specifically due to the use of Allostem or with the harvesting of bone graft from the distal tibia (**Table 1**).

POSTOPERATIVE CARE

Postoperatively, a short leg cast splint was applied. At 2 weeks, the sutures were removed, and the ankle was immobilized in a pneumatic CAM boot for 6 weeks. The patient should remain non-weight-bearing for a total of 6 to 8 weeks.

Nonsteroidal anti-inflammatory and prolonged steroidal drugs were avoided for 12 weeks. Low-dose aspirin for prophylactic anticoagulation, episodic steroid use, and inhaled steroids for asthmatic patients were all acceptable.

Standard weight-bearing radiographs should be done preoperatively and at 6 weeks, 3 months, 6 months, and yearly after the surgery. Radiographs will include 3 views of the ankle. A computed tomography (CT) scan with appropriate axial and coronal cuts will be obtained at 12 weeks. The 3-month radiographs and CT scan will be examined by an independent examiner, who will be masked to the treatment, to determine if arthrodesis is present. The indicators of arthrodesis will be bridging bone across the fused joint, disappearance of the subtalar joint line, and incorporation of the bone graft or new bone adjacent to the subtalar joint on both radiograph and or CT scan.

Table 1		
A comparison of the use of Allostem versus Autograft		
Adverse Event	Allostem (%)	Autograft (%)
Screws removed	19	17
Wound-healing issues	4.3	6.6
Foot pain or peroneal tendonitis	12	10

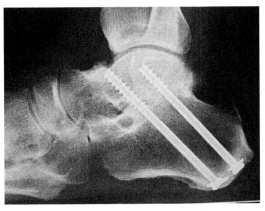

Fig. 2. A case of complete subtalar arthrodesis by radiographs.

OUTCOMES

The authors are in the process of collecting final 2-year data to statistically compare outcome scores (AOFAS, FFI-R and SF-12, VAS) between the 2 groups. In addition, repeated measures analysis of variance will be used to determine significant changes at each time point within groups. Finally, paired samples t tests will be used to analyze the change in dependent variables from preoperative to postoperative (2 years) within each group. One hundred ten patients completed the study.

The exact data are not available for reporting at this point, but the following will probably be confirmed at the conclusion:

- Arthrodesis rates were about the same for both groups.
- There is no statistical difference in any of the outcomes scores.
- Radiographs are of little value to determine whether the subtalar joint is fused.
- CT scan is the most reliable method to evaluate arthrodesis.
- It can take at least 6 months for the subtalar joint to be fused more than 25% of its surface area.
- It is not necessary for the entire subtalar joint to be fused to be pain free (**Figs. 2 and 3**).

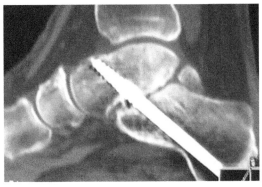

Fig. 3. A case where the arthrodesis looked solid by radiograph, but the CT scan at 6 months showed no arthrodesis.

SUMMARY

No biologic will substitute for poor surgical technique. Diligent joint preparation is critical to success of any fusion. Fusing the posterior facet alone might be sufficient in cases without fixed deformity. Subtalar fusions take a long time to mature, and rehabilitation should be planned accordingly. Allostem apears to be noninferior to autograft for subtalar fusions.

REFERENCES

1. Easley ME, Trnka HJ, Schon LC, et al. Isolated subtalar arthrodesis. J Bone Joint Surg Am 2000;82(5):613–24.
2. DiGiovanni CW, Lin SS, Baumhauer JF, et al, North American Orthopedic Foot and Ankle Study Group. Recombinant human platelet-derived growth factor-BB and beta-tricalcium phosphate (rhPDGF-BB/b-TCP): an alternative to autogenous bone graft. J Bone Joint Surg Am 2013;95:1184–92.
3. Musina RA, Bekchanova ES, Sukhikh GT. Comparison of mesenchymal stem cells obtained from different human tissue. Bull Exp Biol Med 2005;139:504–9.
4. Zuk PA, Zhu M, Ashjian P, et al. Human adipose tissue is a source of multipotent stem cells. Mol Biol Cell 2002;13:4279–95.

Platelet-Rich Plasma and Concentrated Bone Marrow Aspirate in Surgical Treatment for Osteochondral Lesions of the Talus

Youichi Yasui, MD[a,b], Andrew W. Ross, BA[a],
John G. Kennedy, MD, MCh, MMSc, FRCS (Orth)[a,*]

KEYWORDS

- Osteochondral lesions of talus • Platelet-rich plasma • Bone marrow stimulations
- Autologous osteochondral transplantation

KEY POINTS

- Operative treatment can result in nearly 85% success rates in short-term and mid-term outcomes in osteochondral lesions of the talus (OLT); however, the inevitable deterioration of the regenerated or grafted cartilage is now of growing concern.
- Basic science studies have shown that the use of platelet-rich plasma (PRP) and concentrated bone marrow aspirate (CBMA) can improve cartilage repair and the biological environment of the operated ankle joint; however, the clinical use of those biologics in OLT has not been well described to date.
- Bone marrow stimulation produces reparative fibrous cartilage tissue after the debridement of flapped cartilage, necrotic bone, and calcified layer of the talar lesion.
- Autologous autograft transfer is a replacement procedure that uses cylindrical autologous osteochondral graft(s) to fill the talar defect in OLT.
- Currently available basic and clinical evidence suggests that the use of PRP and CBMA as an adjunct to the surgical procedures used to treat OLT can improve clinical and radiological outcomes.

Dr J.G. Kennedy is a consultant for Arteriocyte, Inc; received research support from the Ohnell Family Foundation, Mr. and Mrs. Michael J Levitt, Arteriocyte Inc; is a board member for the European Society of Sports Traumatology, Knee Surgery, and Arthroscopy (ESSKA), International Society for Cartilage Repair of the Ankle (ISCRA), American Orthopedic Foot & Ankle Society (AOFAS) Awards and Scholarships Committee, International Cartilage Repair Society (ICRS) finance board; Drs Y. Yasui and A.W. Ross have nothing to disclose.

[a] The Foot & Ankle Service, Hospital for Special Surgery, 523 East 72nd Street, Suite 507, New York, NY 10021, USA; [b] Department of Orthopaedic Surgery, Teikyo University School of Medicine, 2-11-1 Kaga, Itabashi, Tokyo 173-8605, Japan
* Corresponding author. 523 East 72nd Street, Suite 507, New York, NY 10021.
E-mail address: kennedyj@hss.edu

1083-7515/16/© 2016 Elsevier Inc. All rights reserved.

INTRODUCTION

Osteochondral lesions of the talus (OLT) frequently accompany foot and ankle injuries, including ankle sprains and fractures.[1] When conservative measures fail to relieve a patient's symptoms, operative treatment, including both reparative and replacement techniques, is indicated.[2] Clinical evidence suggests that both operative treatment modalities demonstrate good to excellent short-term and mid-term clinical outcomes in up to 85% of cases.[3] Nevertheless, the technical difficulty of the operative procedures and the inevitable deterioration of the regenerated or grafted cartilage are of concern.[4–7] Previous studies propose that a combination of mechanical and biological impairments in the injured ankle joint may affect the deterioration, prompting interest in adjuvant modalities that could improve outcomes by addressing some of these deficits.

Platelet-rich plasma (PRP) and concentrated bone marrow aspirate (CBMA) are simple, minimally invasive procedures that could potentially improve the quality of cartilage repair and the biological environment in the ankle joint.[8] Despite numerous basic science articles showing evidence of the benefits associated with the use of these biologics for the treatment of cartilage lesions,[2,8–24] the production techniques used to generate these products and the clinical outcomes following their use in conjunction with operative treatment for OLT have not been well described to date.

In this article, we describe the surgical techniques of the 2 most common operative procedures for OLT, bone marrow stimulation (BMS) and autologous autograft transfer (AOT), and present the current evidence on the use of biologic agents in conjunction with the surgical procedures described.

INDICATIONS/CONTRAINDICATIONS

Operative treatment is indicated for patients who do not experience symptom relief after 3 months of conservative treatment. It is generally accepted that BMS is performed on patients with small lesion size, whereas AOT is applied in large defects. Currently, the critical size has been established at 15 mm[25] in a diameter or 150 mm^2.[26,27] Contraindications for surgery include any patient identified as a smoker or having associated medical comorbidities (eg, diabetes, autoimmune disease, active infection). Knee arthritis and patellofemoral syndrome are only relative contraindications for AOT. Global joint degeneration is a controversial indication for BMS, but is contraindicated for AOT. Patients with previous failed BMS may experience better outcomes with AOT.[28]

Indications for use of biologics in both BMS and AOT are not well defined yet in clinical evidence or practice. In the authors' institution, these biologics are not used in patients, with (1) hematologic dyscarsias, particularly platelet dysfunction, (2) active infection, and (3) severe anemia (hemoglobin level <8 g/dL).

Preoperative Planning

In certain cases, the diagnosis of OLT can be challenging due to a lack of specific clinical symptoms indicating the presence of a lesion and possible false-positive interpretation of standard radiographs.[29–32] A high index of doubt is present in cases with persistent ankle pain following ankle injuries.

OLT commonly occurs concomitantly with other ankle pathologies (eg, synovitis, bony spur, ligament injuries). Examination for the presence of these common concomitant pathologies is also evaluated preoperatively.

Imaging studies are used to diagnose OLT and plan the operative treatment. In 30% to 50% of cases, standard radiographs fail to detect OLT.[29–32] Computed tomography

(CT) and MRI are more accurate imaging modalities for identifying OLTs (CT, sensitivity: 0.81, specificity: 0.99; MRI, sensitivity: 0.96, specificity: 0.96).[29]

Lesion size parameters are measured on axial, sagittal, and coronal views on CT and MRI. As mentioned previously, the critical size of 15 mm in diameter or 150 mm^2 determines the surgical modality that is used.[25–27] The authors prefer to measure the longest length of the lesion between the rims of surrounding cartilage layer (**Fig. 1**). Lesion area is calculated according to an established method (diameter $\times$ diameter $\times$ 0.79).[26]

SURGICAL TECHNIQUE/PROCEDURES
Preparation of Biologics

PRP and CBMA are produced according to the guidelines of available commercial systems before the operation.

Platelet-rich plasma

PRP is a simple blood product that contains more than double the concentration of platelets compared with baseline values, or greater than 1.1×10^6 platelets/μL.[8,33]

The plasma is a reservoir of growth factors and cytokines that participate in tissue healing.[8,33]

Basic science in vitro and in vivo studies have shown that PRP has chondrogenic and anti-inflammatory effects.[8,33] PRP may also attract mesenchymal stem cells (MSCs) to the site of their injection.[8,34] Numerous high-level clinical studies support the use of PRP for the treatment for osteoarthritis[14–20,35–37] and a few have examined the effect of PRP in OLT.[21–23,38]

The preparation of PRP consists of 2 steps: (1) venous blood is drawn from a peripheral vein, typically the anterocubital fossa vein. (2) The blood is centrifuged using commercially available PRP centrifuge systems. To date, no standardized PRP production method has been established. Various commercially available PRP centrifuge modalities, timing protocols for the centrifugation of harvested blood, and PRP activation methods have been described.[34,39–41] Due to the diversity of production methods, the contents of the PRP are variable, even within a single individual.[40]

Concentrated bone marrow aspirate

CBMA is blood product similar to PRP that includes abundant MSCs in addition to the growth factors and cytokines found in PRP.[42]

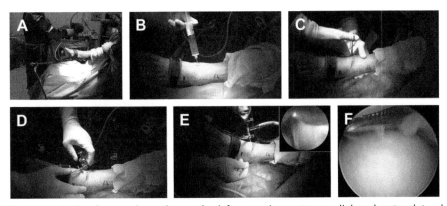

Fig. 1. (*A–F*) The figures show the method for creating anteromedial and anterolateral portals.

CBMA has the potential to improve the quality of cartilage repair tissue. In animal studies, CBMA improved healing compared with BMS alone based on histologic and radiological parameters.[9,24]

CBMA is produced by centrifuging bone marrow aspirate (BMA) harvested from the patient's iliac crest using a trocar at the time of surgery for OLT. BMA can be obtained from various sites, including the iliac crest, greater trochanter, tibia in children, and the sternum, particularly in very obese patients.

OPERATIVE PROCEDURES
Bone Marrow Stimulation

BMS is a reparative procedure that aims to stimulate MSC proliferation and promote the formation of regenerative fibrous cartilage repair tissue in the OLT defect.[2] The procedure can be performed under ankle arthroscopy and is considered minimally invasive.

Preparation and patient positioning
The patient lays supine on the operative table with the hip ipsilateral to the site of the lesion flexed and supported by a well padded leg holder (see **Fig. 1**A). The thigh holder is positioned proximal to the popliteal fossa. This positioning allows neurovascular structures to be protected, which may decrease the risk of DVT.

A thigh tourniquet is applied.

The ankle should be distracted noninvasively using a commercially available, sterile distraction strap. This allows intraoperative ankle joint motion in dorsiflexion and plantar flexion, as well as increases the space within the ankle joint.

Surgical procedure
Step 1: making portals Anteromedial (AM), anterolateral (AL), and occasionally posterolateral (PL) portals are used in BMS.

Before any incisions are made, anatomic landmarks, including the lateral malleoli (LM), medial malleoli (MM), peroneaus tertius, tibialis anterior tendon (TAT), superficial peroneal nerve, and sural nerve are marked. This step is of particular importance, as the highest postoperative complication following ankle arthroscopic procedures is injury to the superficial peroneal nerve, which accounts for up to 2.7% of complications.[11,43]

At the level of ankle joint, the AM portal should be located just medial to the medial border of the TAT and the AL portal is placed lateral to the peroneus tertius. The PL portal is positioned 1.0 mm anterior to the lateral borders of Achilles tendon and at the level of the horizontal lines between the inferior pole of the MM and the tip of LM.

The authors usually make portals in the following order: AM portal, AL portal, and PL portals. "Nick and spread" technique is always used to decrease risk of iatrogenic complications.

AM portal: A 22-gauge needle is inserted from the previously marked AM portal into the ankle joint. Saline is then injected into the ankle (see **Fig. 1**B). After making a skin incision using a #11 blade, subcutaneous blunt dissection is performed using a mosquito clamp (see **Fig. 1**C). A 2.7-mm arthroscope sleeve with a trocar is gently advanced into the ankle joint (see **Fig. 1**D). It is then switched out for a 2.7-mm 30° arthroscope.

AL portal: The needle is inserted from the site of previously marked AL portal into the ankle joint (see **Fig. 1**E). Once the location of the needle is confirmed under arthroscopy, the superficial incision and subcutaneous blunt dissection are performed (see **Fig. 1**F).

PL portal: This portal is occasionally used to better visualize the posterior aspect of the ankle joint. The approach is just lateral to the lateral border of the Achilles tendon with care taken to avoid the sural nerve. The PL portal is created in a fashion similar to that described previously using a "nick and spread" technique.

Step 2: diagnostic examination within the ankle joint Intra-articular structures should be reviewed systematically using the "21 points examination."[44]

The margins of the OLT are identified using the probe.

OLT frequently accompanies concomitant ankle pathologies (eg, synovitis, bony spur, ligament injuries). These lesions can be treated at the same time that BMS is performed.

Step 3: debridement of unstable cartilage, necrotic bone, and calcified layer Flapped cartilage, necrotic bone, and calcified layer are debrided using an angled curette and a motorized suction shaver (**Fig. 2**A). It is important to confirm the stable rim of remaining cartilage. Failure to excise loose fragments and dead cartilage will lead to failure of the surgical procedure.[45]

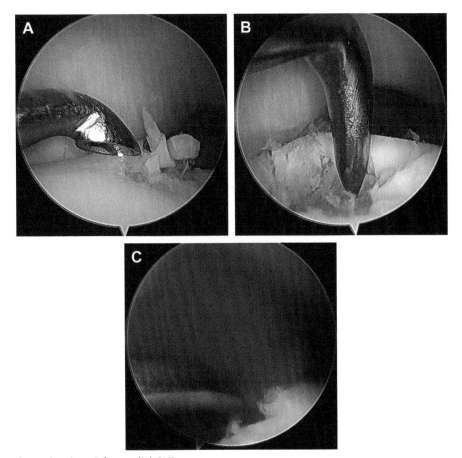

Fig. 2. (*A–C*) BMS for medial OLT.

Avoid iatrogenic cartilage damage by using multiple specialized instruments and changing portals for best visualization. In ankle arthroscopy, iatrogenic cartilage damage is not rare (up to 31%).[46]

Step 4: penetrating the subchondral bone plate Microfracture/drilling using microfracture pick/drill is performed to penetrate the subchondral bone plate (**Fig. 2B**). The holes are spaced approximately 4 mm apart and drilled to a depth of approximately 3 mm.

The sensation accompanying penetration of the subchondral bone plate can be described as drilling "from hard to soft."

Blood from the created holes can be observed when inflow pressure is decreased and is used to confirm that appropriate drilling depth has been reached.

Outcomes following BMS of uncontained lesions are inferior to those of contained lesions.[27] The BMS technique for uncontained lesions and contained lesions is similar. No dead cartilage or bone should be left in site.

Step 5: biologics PRP and CBMA are injected into the bed of the lesion following a water-tight closure (**Fig. 2C**).

Biologics are also injected into the joint following wound closure.

Postoperative management
Sutures are usually removed 7 to 10 days postoperatively.

Active range of motion exercises are encouraged as soon as possible.

The patient is non–weight-bearing for the first 2 weeks following surgery, partially weight-bearing for an 2 additional weeks, and then full weight-bearing at 4 weeks postoperatively.

Potential complications
Although ankle arthroscopic procedures are minimally invasive, up to 9% of patients report postoperative complications.[10,11,27,43,44,47–49] The superficial peroneal nerve is the most commonly injured nerve during arthroscopic ankle procedures.[9,11,43,50–52]

One clinical study reported that iatrogenic cartilage damage following ankle arthroscopy using mainly 4.0-mm arthroscopy is extremely high (31% overall, superficial lesion: 24.3%, severe lesion: 6.7%).[46]

Reparative fibrous cartilage inevitably deteriorates over time.[4–7,53]

Outcomes
Bone marrow stimulation Approximately 85% of patients have successful clinical outcomes.[3,54,55]

Approximately 90% athletes return to full sports activities.[56,57]

Bone marrow stimulation with biologics Currently, only 4 comparative studies (BMS with/without biologics) have been published.

Guney and colleagues[22,38]: a randomized prospective study. Compared 16 patients who received BMS alone were compared with 19 patients who received both BMS and PRP. At the average follow-up of 16.2 months, all cases had significantly improved clinical outcomes, but the BMS + PRP group had better outcomes compared with the BMS-only group.

Another Guney and collegues[38]: comparative study. Nineteen patients who received BMS were compared with 22 patients who received BMS and PRP and 13 patients who received mosaicplasty. At an average of 42-month follow-up, all groups had significantly improved clinical outcomes.

Görmeli and colleagues[23]: a prospective randomized clinical trial. Thirteen patients who received BMS and saline were compared with 14 patients who received BMS and hyaluronic acid (HA) and 13 patients who received BMS and PRP. At an average of 15.3-month follow-up, clinical improvement following the addition of PRP to BMS was significantly greater than after HA or saline injection.

Hannon and colleagues[58]: a retrospective comparative study. Twelve patients who received BMS alone were compared with 22 patients who received BMS and CBMA. BMS with CBMA resulted in comparably good medium-term functional outcomes, but improved border repair tissue and showed less evidence of cartilage fissuring and fibrillation on MRI compared with BMS alone.

Autologous Osteochondral Transplantation

AOT is a replacement procedure for OLT in which the lesion is filled with cylindrical autologous osteochondral graft(s), typically from a non–weight-bearing portion of the ipsilateral femoral condyle.[2,59] In AOT, the surface of the graft must be aligned precisely with the native cartilage surface, necessitating grafts that are of equal height to the depth of the defect.[2,59] Step off between graft and surrounding tissue is not acceptable and could lead to poor surgical outcomes in the joint.[60]

Preparation and patient positioning

The patient lays supine on the operating table and a thigh tourniquet is applied.

Surgical procedure

Step 1: tibial osteotomy to provide visualization of osteochondral lesions of the talus The purpose of the osteotomy is to create a direct path for inserting the osteochondral graft into the site of the OLT. In AOT, it is essential to reconstruct a smooth articular surface. Patients with lesions located on the anterior aspect of talus can be treated via arthroscopic or mini-open approach without the need for an osteotomy. However, when the surgeon cannot obtain a perpendicular view with medial or lateral lesions, a medial malleolar or trapezoidal osteotomy should be performed to create optimal access to the lesion.[61]

Medial osteochondral lesions of the talus: a chevron osteotomy A longitudinal skin incision line is marked over the medial malleolus. The skin is cut using a #15 blade, with care to protect the great saphenous nerve.

The medial corner of anterior aspect of the tibia and the posteromedial aspect of the tibia are exposed.

A Kirschner (K) wire is inserted from the medial aspect of the tibia to direct to medical corner of ankle joint under fluoroscopic guidance (**Fig. 3**A). The tip of the K-wire should be in the tibia to avoid additional damage to the cartilage.

To prepare for a chevron-type osteotomy, the periosteum is reflected back from the apex (K-wire insertion point) to the anteromedial/posteromedial corner of the ankle joint. The posterior tibialis tendon must be protected to avoid iatrogenic damage.

Two parallel fixation holes are predrilled in the medial malleolus before the osteotomy (**Fig. 3**B).

A chevron-type osteotomy is performed using a bone saw and osteotome. This should be done with caution to avoid damage to the neurovascular bundle as well as the posterior tibialis tendon (**Fig. 3**C).

Lateral lesion: a trapezoidal osteotomy A lateral tibial trapezoidal osteotomy can be made to provide access to all but the most posterior lesions, thereby avoiding fibular takedown.[62]

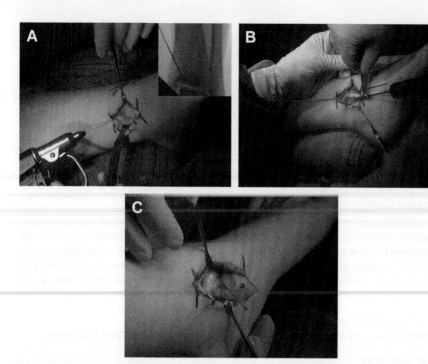

Fig. 3. (*A–C*) A chevron osteotomy. [a] Medial malleolus.

A longitudinal incision line is marked lateral to the extensor digitorum longus. The skin is cut using a #15 blade.

Careful to protect branches of the superficial peroneal nerve (**Fig. 4**A), the soft tissue under the skin is dissected to expose the anterior aspect of the tibia.

One fixation hole is predrilled in the anterior aspect of the tibia before the osteotomy (**Fig. 4**B).

A trapezoidal osteotomy is performed using a bone saw and osteotome (**Fig. 4**C).

Step 2: removing the lesion from the talus, bone marrow stimulation, and overdrill The lesion, including damaged cartilage and bone, is removed using a commercially available trephine with controlled taps of mallet to a depth of 10 mm (**Fig. 5**A, B).

BMS is performed in the surrounding healthy bone from the medial wall of the recipient site that has been created (**Fig. 5**C).

The recipient site is deepened to make a hole slightly deeper than harvested graft (**Fig. 5**D).

Step 3: harvest osteochondral graft from a non–weight-bearing portion of the ipsilateral femoral condyle A mini-arthrotomy along the lateral border of the patella is performed to access the lateral femoral condyle (**Fig. 6**A).

Osteochondral graft(s) from a non–weight-bearing portion of the knee are harvested using a commercially available trephine, with extra care to position the harvester correctly (**Fig. 6**B). The harvester should be perpendicular to the joint surface, ensuring the topography of the graft is optimally matched with the talar dome.

The length of the graft is approximately 10 mm (**Fig. 6**C).

Step 4: the graft or grafts are transferred into the created recipient site A rongeur is used to shape the end of the graft to allow improved seating during press-fit insertion.

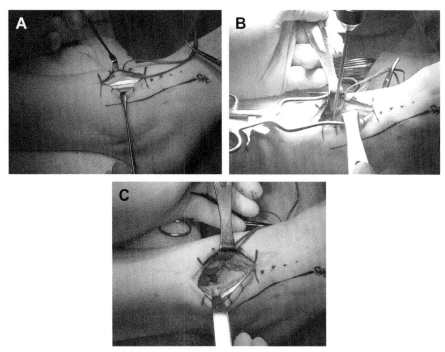

Fig. 4. (*A–C*) A trapezoidal osteotomy.

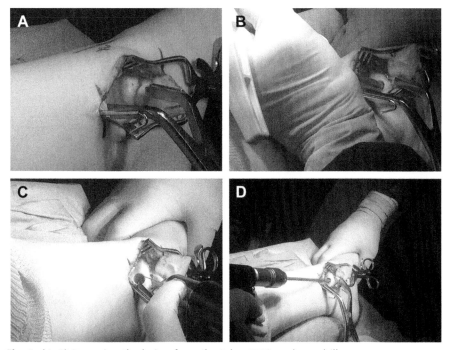

Fig. 5. (*A–D*) Removing the lesion from the talus, BMS, and overdrill.

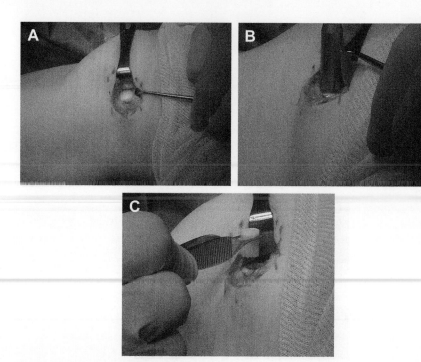

Fig. 6. (*A–C*) Harvest osteochondral graft.

The osteochondral graft is bathed in the PRP or CBMA before insertion.

Then, 1.0 mL of CBMA and PRP are injected into the created recipient site.

The osteochondral graft is inserted into the recipient site. The highest part of the graft and the talus should be aligned to ensure anatomic congruency in the vertical plan, forming a flat articular surface (**Fig. 7**). However, a biomechanical study demonstrates an acceptable range between 1 mm sunken to 0.4 mm proud (see **Fig. 7**).[16]

Step 5: fixation of medial malleolus In the medial tibial osteotomy, the fragment is reduced anatomically and fixed using 3 screws (**Fig. 8**).

In the lateral tibial osteotomy, a single predrilled 4-mm titanium screw is used for final fixation of the osteotomy.

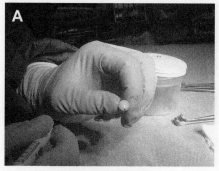
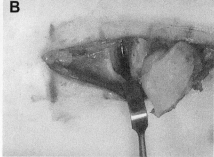

Fig. 7. (*A, B*) Insertion of graft.

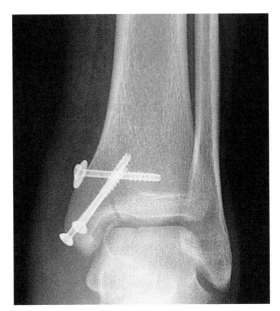

Fig. 8. Postoperative radiograph of medial OLT.

Step 6: biologics To promote a systemic or trophic effect on the synovium and sur-rounding cartilage after wound closure, 2.0 mL of CBMA or PRP is injected into the ankle joint.

Postoperative management
Sutures are usually removed 10 to 14 days postoperatively.

The ankle is immobilized in a short-leg splint for 2 weeks following surgery, replaced with a CAM boot for 4 additional weeks. Bony union of the osteotomy site is usually achieved 6 weeks after surgery.

Active range of motion exercises are encouraged as soon as possible after removal of the splint.

After the splint is removed, the patient is non–weight-bearing for first 2 weeks, 10% weight-bearing for the following 2 weeks, and increasing weight until full weight-bearing is achieved in the 2 weeks following.

Potential complications
Possible mal/nonunion and degenerative change at the site of osteotomy.[63]

Knee pain.[64]

Poor integration of the graft at the interface between the implanted osteochondral graft and surrounding tissue.[65,66]

Cyst formation around the osteochondral graft.[64]

Outcomes
Autologous osteochondral transplantation Nearly 90% good to excellent outcomes following AOT.[3]

Sixty-three percent to 95% of athletes return to full activity.[10,11,67,68]

Autologous osteochondral transplantation with biologics Currently, AOT supple-mented with biologic agents is a novel technique. Therefore, basic science and clinical evidence on outcomes associated with this modality are very limited.

Smyth and colleagues[12]: comparative study in a rabbit osteochondral lesion model. Found that application of PRP at the time of AOT improved the integration of the osteochondral graft at the cartilage interface and decreased graft degeneration.

Boakye and colleagues[13]: comparative study in a rabbit osteochondral lesion model. Showed that transforming growth factor-β1 expression was increased in rabbits treated with AOT and PRP compared with those treated with AOT and saline, concluding that PRP may have a chondrogenic effect in vivo.

Kennedy and Murawsk[10]: A single report on CBMA in OLT patients treated with AOT. Showed significant improvement of clinical outcomes in 72 patients at a mean follow-up of 28 months. In addition, the investigators reported that MRI using T2 mapping showed restoration of radius curvature and color stratification similar to that of native cartilage.

SUMMARY

OLT is a common orthopedic disorder. Despite high success rates following reparative and placement procedures, postoperative deterioration of the operated ankle joint over time is inevitable. Currently available basic and clinical studies suggest that the biologic agents PRP and CBMA can improve the clinical and radiological outcomes in OLT when used in conjunction with surgical modalities. However, room exists for continued development, improvement, and standardization of these techniques. Thus, further well-designed clinical trials establishing the utility of biologics in the treatment of OLT are warranted.

REFERENCES

1. Guillo S, Bauer T, Lee JW, et al. Consensus in chronic ankle instability: aetiology, assessment, surgical indications and place for arthroscopy. Orthop Traumatol Surg Res 2013;99(8 Suppl):S411–9.
2. Murawski CD, Kennedy JG. Operative treatment of osteochondral lesions of the talus. J Bone Joint Surg Am 2013;95(11):1045–54.
3. Zengerink M, Struijs PA, Tol JL, et al. Treatment of osteochondral lesions of the talus: a systematic review. Knee Surg Sports Traumatol Arthrosc 2010;18(2): 238–46.
4. Robinson DE, Winson IG, Harries WJ, et al. Arthroscopic treatment of osteochondral lesions of the talus. J Bone Joint Surg Br 2003;85(7):989–93.
5. Ferkel RD, Zanotti RM, Komenda GA, et al. Arthroscopic treatment of chronic osteochondral lesions of the talus: long-term results. Am J Sports Med 2008;36(9): 1750–62.
6. Lee KB, Bai LB, Yoon TR, et al. Second-look arthroscopic findings and clinical outcomes after microfracture for osteochondral lesions of the talus. Am J Sports Med 2009;37(1):63S–70S.
7. Becher C, Driessen A, Hess T, et al. Microfracture for chondral defects of the talus: maintenance of early results at midterm follow-up. Knee Surg Sports Traumatol Arthrosc 2010;18(5):656–63.
8. Smyth NA, Murawski CD, Fortier LA, et al. Platelet-rich plasma in the pathologic processes of cartilage: review of basic science evidence. Arthroscopy 2013; 29(8):1399–409.
9. Fortier LA, Potter HG, Rickey EJ, et al. Concentrated bone marrow aspirate improves full-thickness cartilage repair compared with microfracture in the equine model. J Bone Joint Surg Am 2010;92-A:1927–37.

10. Kennedy J, Murawsk C. The treatment of osteochondral lesions of the talus with autologous osteochondral transplantation and bone marrow aspirate concentrate: surgical technique. Cartilage 2011;2(4):327–36.
11. Fraser EJ, Harris MC, Prado MP, et al. Autologous osteochondral transplantation for osteochondral lesions of the talus in an athletic population. Knee Surg Sports Traumatol Arthrosc 2016;24(4):1272–9.
12. Smyth NA, Haleem AM, Murawski CD, et al. The effect of platelet-rich plasma on autologous osteochondral transplantation: an in vivo rabbit model. J Bone Joint Surg Am 2013;95(24):2185–93.
13. Boakye LA, Ross KA, Pinski JM, et al. Platelet-rich plasma increases transforming growth factor-beta1 expression at graft-host interface following autologous osteochondral transplantation in a rabbit model. World J Orthop 2015;6(11):961–9.
14. Raeissadat SA, Rayegani SM, Hassanabadi H, et al. Knee osteoarthritis injection choices: platelet- rich plasma (PRP) versus hyaluronic acid (a one-year randomized clinical trial). Clin Med Insights Arthritis Musculoskelet Disord 2015;8:1–8.
15. Rayegani SM, Raeissadat SA, Taheri MS, et al. Does intra articular platelet rich plasma injection improve function, pain and quality of life in patients with osteoarthritis of the knee? A randomized clinical trial. Orthop Rev (Pavia) 2014;6(3):5405.
16. Battaglia M, Guaraldi F, Vannini F, et al. Efficacy of ultrasound-guided intra-articular injections of platelet-rich plasma versus hyaluronic acid for hip osteoarthritis. Orthopedics 2013;36(12):e1501–8.
17. Manunta AF, Manconi A. The treatment of chondral lesions of the knee with the microfracture technique and platelet-rich plasma. Joints 2014;1(4):167–70.
18. Patel S, Dhillon MS, Aggarwal S, et al. Treatment with platelet-rich plasma is more effective than placebo for knee osteoarthritis: a prospective, double-blind, randomized trial. Am J Sports Med 2013;41(2):356–64.
19. Filardo G, Kon E, Di Martino A, et al. Platelet-rich plasma vs hyaluronic acid to treat knee degenerative pathology: study design and preliminary results of a randomized controlled trial. BMC Musculoskelet Disord 2012;13:229.
20. Cerza F, Carnì S, Carcangiu A, et al. Comparison between hyaluronic acid and platelet-rich plasma, intra-articular infiltration in the treatment of gonarthrosis. Am J Sports Med 2012;40(12):2822–7.
21. Mei-Dan O, Carmont MR, Laver L, et al. Platelet-rich plasma or hyaluronate in the management of osteochondral lesions of the talus. Am J Sports Med 2012;40:534–41.
22. Guney A, Akar M, Karaman I, et al. Clinical outcomes of platelet rich plasma (PRP) as an adjunct to microfracture surgery in osteochondral lesions of the talus. Knee Surg Sports Traumatol Arthrosc 2015;23(8):2384–9.
23. Görmeli G, Karakaplan M, Görmeli CA, et al. Clinical effects of platelet-rich plasma and hyaluronic acid as an additional therapy for talar osteochondral lesions treated with microfracture surgery: a prospective randomized clinical trial. Foot Ankle Int 2015;36(8):891–900.
24. Saw KY, Hussin P, Loke SC, et al. Articular cartilage regeneration with autologous marrow aspirate and hyaluronic acid: an experimental study in a goat model. Arthroscopy 2009;25(12):1391–400.
25. Chuckpaiwong B, Berkson EM, Theodore GH. Microfracture for osteochondral lesions of the ankle: outcome analysis and outcome predictors of 105 cases. Arthroscopy 2008;24(1):106–12.
26. Choi WJ, Park KK, Kim BS, et al. Osteochondral lesion of the talus: is there a critical defect size for poor outcome? Am J Sports Med 2009;37(10):1974–80.

27. Choi WJ, Choi GW, Kim JS, et al. Prognostic significance of the containment and location of osteochondral lesions of the talus: independent adverse outcomes associated with uncontained lesions of the talar shoulder. Am J Sports Med 2013;41(1):126–33.

28. Ross AW, Murawski CD, Fraser EJ, et al. Autologous osteochondral transplantation for osteochondral lesions of the talus: does previous bone marrow stimulation negatively affect clinical outcome? Arthroscopy 2016;32(7):1377–83.

29. Verhagen RA, Maas M, Dijkgraff MG, et al. Prospective study on diagnostic strategies in osteochondral lesions of the talus. Is MRI superior to helical CT? J Bone Joint Surg Br 2005;87:41–6.

30. Hepple S, Winson IG, Glew D. Osteochondral lesions of the talus: a revised classification. Foot Ankle Int 1999;20:789–93.

31. Flick AB, Gould N. Osteochondritis dissecans of the talus (transchondral fractures of the talus): review of the literature and new surgical approach for medial dome lesions. Foot Ankle 1993;21:13–9.

32. Loomer R, Fischer C, Lloyd-Smith R, et al. Osteochondral lesions of the talus. Am J Sports Med 1984;12:460–3.

33. Boswell SG, Cole BJ, Sundman EA, et al. Platelet rich plasma: a milieu of bioactive factors. Arthroscopy 2012;28(3):429–39.

34. Holmes HL, Wilson B, Silverberg JL, et al. Identification of the optimal biologic to enhance endogenous stem cell recruitment. ORS. Annual Meeting. New Orleans, Louisiana, March 15-18, 2014.

35. Meheux CJ, McCulloch PC, Lintner DM, et al. Efficacy of intra-articular platelet-rich plasma injections in knee osteoarthritis: a systematic review. Arthroscopy 2016;32(3):495–505.

36. Riboh JC, Saltzman BM, Yanke AB, et al. Effect of leukocyte concentration on the efficacy of platelet-rich plasma in the treatment of knee osteoarthritis. Am J Sports Med 2016;44(3):792–800.

37. Laudy AB, Bakker EW, Rekers M, et al. Efficacy of platelet-rich plasma injections in osteoarthritis of the knee: a systematic review and meta-analysis. Br J Sports Med 2015;49(10):657–72.

38. Guney A, Yurdakul E, Karaman I, et al. Medium-term outcomes of mosaicplasty versus arthroscopic microfracture with or without platelet-rich plasma in the treatment of osteochondral lesions of the talus. Knee Surg Sports Traumatol Arthrosc 2016;24(4):1293–8.

39. Chubinskaya S, Huch K, Mikecz K, et al. Chondrocyte matrix metalloproteinase-8: up-regulation of neutrophil collagenase by interleukin-1 beta in human cartilage from knee and ankle joints. Lab Invest 1996;74(1):232–40.

40. Sundman EA, Cole BJ, Fortier LA. Growth factor and catabolic cytokine concentrations are influenced by the cellular composition of platelet-rich plasma. Am J Sports Med 2011;39(10):2135–40.

41. Davis VL, Abukabda AB, Radio NM, et al. Platelet-rich preparations to improve healing. Part II: platelet activation and enrichment, leukocyte inclusion, and other selection criteria. J Oral Implantol 2014;40(4):511–21.

42. Cassano JM, Kennedy JG, Ross KA, et al. Bone marrow concentrate and platelet-rich plasma differ in cell distribution and interleukin 1 receptor antagonist protein concentration. Knee Surg Sports Traumatol Arthrosc 2016. [Epub ahead of print].

43. Adams SB, Setton LA, Bell RD, et al. Inflammatory cytokines and matrix metalloproteinases in the synovial fluid after intra-articular ankle fracture. Foot Ankle Int 2015;36(11):1264–71.

44. Ferkel RD, Fischer SP. Progress in ankle arthroscopy. Clin Orthop Relat Res 1989; 240:210–20.
45. Takao M, Uchio Y, Kakimaru H, et al. Arthroscopic drilling with debridement of remaining cartilage for osteochondral lesions of the talar dome in unstable ankles. Am J Sports Med 2004;32(2):332–6.
46. Vega J, Golanó P, Peña F. Iatrogenic articular cartilage injuries during ankle arthroscopy. Knee Surg Sports Traumatol Arthrosc 2016;24(4):1304–10.
47. Simonson DC, Roukis TS. Safety of ankle arthroscopy for the treatment of anterolateral soft-tissue impingement. Arthroscopy 2014;30(2):256–9.
48. van Dijk CN, van Bergen CJ. Advancements in ankle arthroscopy. J Am Acad Orthop Surg 2008;16(11):635–46.
49. Zwiers R, Wiegerinck JI, Murawski CD, et al. Arthroscopic treatment for anterior ankle impingement: a systematic review of the current literature. Arthroscopy 2015;31(8):1585–96.
50. Freed LE, Marquis JC, Nohria A, et al. Neocartilage formation in vitro and in vivo using cells cultured on synthetic biodegradable polymers. J Biomed Mater Res 1993;27(1):11–23.
51. van Susante JL, Buma P, van Osch GJ, et al. Culture of chondrocytes in alginate and collagen carrier gels. Acta Orthop Scand 1995;66(6):549–56.
52. Grigolo B, Lisignoli G, Piacentini A, et al. Evidence for redifferentiation of human chondrocytes grown on a hyaluronan-based biomaterial (HYAff 11): molecular, immunohistochemical and ultrastructural analysis. Biomaterials 2002;23(4): 1187–95.
53. Polat G, Erşen A, Erdil ME, et al. Long-term results of microfracture in the treatment of talus osteochondral lesions. Knee Surg Sports Traumatol Arthrosc 2016;24(4):1299–303.
54. Tol JL, Struijs PA, Bossuyt PM, et al. Treatment strategies in osteochondral defects of the talar dome: a systematic review [Review]. Foot Ankle Int 2000; 21(2):119–26.
55. Verhagen RA, Struijs PA, Bossuyt PM, et al. Systematic review of treatment strategies for osteochondral defects of the talar dome. Foot Ankle Clin 2003;8(2): 233–42, viii-ix.
56. Saxena A, Eakin C. Articular talar injuries in athletes: results of microfracture and autogenous bone graft. Am J Sports Med 2007;35(10):1680–7.
57. van Bergen CJ, Kox LS, Maas M, et al. Arthroscopic treatment of osteochondral defects of the talus: outcomes at eight to twenty years of follow-up. J Bone Joint Surg Am 2013;95(6):519–25.
58. Hannon CP, Ross KA, Murawski CD, et al. Arthroscopic bone marrow stimulation and concentrated bone marrow aspirate for osteochondral lesions of the talus: a case-control study of functional and magnetic resonance observation of cartilage repair tissue outcomes. Arthroscopy 2016;32(2):339–47.
59. Flynn S, Ross KA, Hannon CP, et al. Autologous osteochondral transplantation for osteochondral lesions of the talus. Foot Ankle Int 2016;37(4):363–72.
60. Fansa AM, Murawski CD, Imhauser CW, et al. Autologous osteochondral transplantation of the talus partially restores contact mechanics of the ankle joint. Am J Sports Med 2011;39(11):2457–65.
61. Lee JW. Osteochondral lesions of the talar dome: osteochondral autologous transplantation technique. In: Stone JW, Kennedy JG, Glazebrook MA, editors. The foot and ankle: AANA advanced arthroscopic surgical techniques. Thorofare (NJ): Slack; 2016. p. 19–26.

62. Gianakos AL, Hannon CP, Ross KA, et al. Anterolateral tibial osteotomy for accessing osteochondral lesions of the talus in autologous osteochondral transplantation: functional and t2 MRI analysis. Foot Ankle Int 2015;36(5):531–8.
63. Lamb J, Murawski CD, Deyer TW, et al. Chevron-type medial malleolar osteotomy: a functional, radiographic and quantitative T2-mapping MRI analysis. Knee Surg Sports Traumatol Arthrosc 2013;21(6):1283–8.
64. Valderrabano V, Leumann A, Rasch H, et al. Knee-to-ankle mosaicplasty for the treatment of osteochondral lesions of the ankle joint. Am J Sports Med 2009; 37(Suppl 1):105S–11S.
65. Siebert CH, Miltner O, Weber M, et al. Healing of osteochondral grafts in an ovine model under the influence of bFGF. Arthroscopy 2003;19(2):182–7.
66. Tibesku CO, Daniilidis K, Szuwart T, et al. Influence of hepatocyte growth factor on autologous osteochondral transplants in an animal model. Arch Orthop Trauma Surg 2011;131(8):1145–51.
67. Paul J, Sagstetter M, Lämmle L, et al. Sports activity after osteochondral transplantation of the talus. Am J Sports Med 2012;40(4):870–4.
68. Hangody L, Dobos J, Balo E, et al. Clinical experiences with autologous osteochondral mosaicplasty in an athletic population: a 17-year prospective multicenter study. Am J Sports Med 2010;38(6):1125–33.

Mesenchymal Stem Cell–Bearing Sutures for Tendon Repair and Healing in the Foot and Ankle

Eric W. Tan, MD[a], Lew C. Schon, MD[b],*

KEYWORDS

- Stem cell–bearing suture • Mesenchymal stem cells • Bone marrow

KEY POINTS

- Biological augmentation may be an avenue to improve the structure, organization, and composition of healing tendons.
- The use of mesenchymal stem cell-bearing sutures may serve to increase early tendon strength, augment regeneration of normal tendon, and decrease the overall healing time, all of which should improve clinical outcomes.
- Mesenchymal stem cells appear to remain locally at the repair site and enhance the histologic repair quality of the tendon collagen.

INTRODUCTION

Repair, reconstruction, and transfer of tendons remain continued challenges for the foot and ankle surgeon. Although our surgical interventions have advanced and developed, tendon healing remains a slow, complex process that results in weaker mechanical properties, which may lead to poor functional outcomes and necessitate revision procedures.[1,2]

Tendon healing occurs in 3 distinct, but overlapping, phases: inflammatory, proliferative, and remodeling.[3] Early healing in the inflammatory phase is mediated by the phagocytosis of necrotic materials by macrophages, initiation of angiogenesis, and recruitment of inflammatory cells. Tenocytes migrate to the wound and begin forming type III collagen, which typically lasts for 2 to 3 days. The proliferative phase,

Disclosure: Dr L.C. Schon is coinventor of a stem cell–bearing suture discussed in this review. He is cofounder of Bioactive Surgical Inc and Stem Cell Surgical, LLC and holds stock in both companies. He is also a consultant to Celling Bioscience (Spinesmith) and Zimmer Biomet Biologics. Dr E.W. Tan has nothing to disclose.

[a] Department of Orthopaedic Surgery, Keck School of Medicine, University of Southern California, 1520 San Pablo Street, Suite 2000, Los Angeles, CA 90033, USA; [b] Department of Orthopaedic Surgery, MedStar Union Memorial Hospital, 3333 North Calvert Street, Suite 400, Baltimore, MD 21218, USA
* Corresponding author.
E-mail address: lyn.camire@medstar.net

1083-7515/16/© 2016 Elsevier Inc. All rights reserved.
foot.theclinics.com

which lasts for a few weeks, is marked by the peak synthesis of type III collagen and increased cellularity of the repaired tissues. In the early phase of remodeling, the consolidation stage, the repair tissues become more fibrous and begin to align in the direction of stress. Increased type I collagen is produced, which typically occurs from 6 to 10 weeks. Finally, the maturation stage of remodeling occurs, in which the fibrous tissues become scarlike tendon tissue over the course of 1 year.

The ideal postoperative rehabilitation protocol revolves around a complex and delicate balance between immobilization and motion. Early postoperative motion is recommended not only to reduce the risk of adhesions but also to increase collagen synthesis and improve fiber alignment, which results in higher tensile strength.[4–6] However, early mobilization may be associated with detrimental effects, including gap formation at the repair site and subsequent tendon elongation, which would result in both a delay in healing and decrease in tensile strength.[7,8] In general, tendon repairs seem to be weakest between 5 and 21 days postoperatively.

The crux of the rehabilitation paradox, therefore, lies in strengthening the tendon at the time of the initial repair and early postoperative period. The development of stronger suture materials, increased number of core strands, and improved suture configurations has resulted in improved tendon repair strength.[9,10] With the recent advances in the understanding and application of biologics in orthopedic surgery, biological augmentation may be an avenue to improve the structure, organization, and composition of healing tendons.

Mesenchymal stem cells (MSCs) are pluripotent, self-renewing cells that play a key role in promoting healing.[11,12] MSCs not only release growth factors and cytokines and recruit additional stem cells but also have the capacity to differentiate into osteocytes, chondrocytes, adipocytes, and tenocytes. In addition, MSCs can be harvested with less invasive procedures, are rapidly propagated, and demonstrate low immunogenicity.[13,14] Therefore, the use of MSCs may serve to increase early tendon strength, augment regeneration of normal tendon, and decrease the overall healing time, all of which should improve clinical outcomes.

The use of a suture as a carrier system for the local delivery of MSCs represents an emerging field of research and innovation. It combines the conventional mechanical strength of a suture repair with the potential for promoting additional biological healing. Two types of stem cell sutures have been previously described. Stems cells have been either coated on the exterior of the suture[15] or placed within an inner core of a proprietary braided suture (Stem Cell Suture, Stem Cell Surgical, LLC, Clarksville, MD[16]). In the exterior coating system used by Yao and colleagues,[15] the stem cells are cultured onto the suture over a 1- to 2-week period. In the proprietary method used in Adams and colleagues,[16] a high concentration of cells is sequestered inside a braided matrix, yielding a significantly higher dosage and protecting the cells during suture introduction. The Food and Drug Administration has not cleared either suture types.

INDICATIONS AND CONTRAINDICATIONS

Sutures loaded with MSCs seek to combine the benefits of biological healing augmentation with mechanical stabilization. MSC-bearing sutures are indicated in all situations that sutures are traditionally used. Examples include, but are not limited to, injuries to ligaments and tendons. Any procedure that involves soft tissue repair and fascial closure would potentially benefit from the addition of biological augmentation through MSCs.

Braided sutures are generally contraindicated in wounds that are contaminated or actively infected. However, data exist in the literature that suggest that MSC can exhibit antimicrobial properties.[17]

Furthermore, a conservative approach would also be to specify active cancer as a contraindication, though there is also uncertainty as to whether MSC signaling will stimulate cancer cells or, alternatively, promote an immune response to cancer cells.

POTENTIAL RISKS

Despite the potential benefits associated with stem cells, there are also possible risks, albeit more theoretic than actually reported in the literature, that should be considered. One major issue is the inability to control the migration and differentiation of the locally delivered stem cells. This migration has been reported in several articles when looking at direct injection using a hypodermic needle.[18] Introduction of the cells in conjunction with a scaffold, such as a suture, may limit the dispersion of the cells and might be anticipated to retain the cells more in the area of desired effect.

Although no conclusive data are currently available in the literature, there are concerns that introduction of high concentrations of stem cells may result in ectopic tissue formation, hypertrophy of the target and surrounding tissues, and the risk of tumor formation. In addition, allogenic stem cells may have an increased risk of a foreign-body reaction and graft-versus-host response once they start to differentiate and potentially lose their immune privilege.

Furthermore, the harvest of autologous stem cells does require a separate incision and procedure, which may be associated with minor donor-site pain or wound complications.

OUTCOMES

Currently, a limited number of published animal studies have examined the efficacy of MSC-bearing sutures. No clinical studies have been previously performed.

Using matched pairs of Achilles tendon transections in 105 rats, Yao and colleagues[19] examined the histologic and biomechanical effect of suture externally coated with bone marrow–derived stem cells. When compared with repairs performed with suture without MSCs, tendon repairs using the stem cell–coated suture demonstrated statistically significant greater strength at 7 and 10 days. No significant differences were observed between the two groups at 14 and 28 days. In addition, the stem cells loaded onto the suture were found at the repair site at all time points. Furthermore, there were no macroscopic differences in tendon morphology observed between groups.

Adams and colleagues[16] randomized 108 Achilles transections from 54 rats into 3 repair groups: suture only, suture with local injection of MSCs, and suture loaded with MSCs within the core. The comparison with both a conventional repair and a conventional repair with local injection of MSCs provides important insight into the value of the suture scaffold to the desired result (**Table 1**). Ultimate failure strength was significantly higher in both suture groups supplemented with MSCs compared with the repairs performed with suture alone. Repairs performed with the suture with local injections of MSCs demonstrated a significant decrease in ultimate failure load at 28 days compared with 14 days. However, this decrease was not found in the MSC-loaded suture repair group. Histologic analysis of the tissue revealed significantly better collagen orientation and fewer fibroblasts in the repairs performed with the MSC-loaded sutures compared with the other two groups.

Table 1
Comparison of ultimate failure load, cross-sectional area, and histology data between groups and at 14 versus 28 days

Measurement	Day	Suture Only		Suture + Injection		Suture + MSCs		P Value	
		n	Mean ± SE	n	Mean ± SE	n	Mean ± SE	Group	Time
Ultimate failure load (N/mm²)	14	13	1.3 ± 0.4	10	3.0 ± 1.8	12	3.2 ± 2.6	≤.001ᵃ	.02ᵇ
	28	13	1.3 ± 0.4	12	1.6 ± 0.8	11	2.3 ± 0.8	—	—
Cross-sectional area (mm²)	14	13	18.8 ± 1.4	10	9.7 ± 1.6	12	8.2 ± 1.4	.14	.52
	28	13	18.3 ± 1.1	12	14.8 ± 1.6	11	9.0 ± 0.9	—	—
Histology	14	6	2.7 ± 0.3	7	2.5 ± 0.3	6	1.4 ± 0.1	≤.001ᶜ	.01ᵈ
	28	6	3.39 ± 0.2	6	2.83 ± 0.3	6	2.06 ± 0.1	—	—

Multifactor analysis of variance and Tukey post hoc test were used.

[a] Suture + injection and suture + MSCs were significantly higher than the suture-only group.

[b] A subsequent detailed comparison found that the significant decrease in failure strength over time was primarily attributed to the suture + injection group ($P = .02$). Suture only, $P = .82$; suture + MSCs, $P = .26$.

[c] Suture + MSCs was significantly lower (better) than suture-only and suture + injection groups.

[d] Histology score was significantly higher (poorer) at 28 days than at 14 days for all groups.

From Adams SB Jr, Thorpe MA, Parks BG, et al. Stem cell cell-bearing suture improves achilles tendon healing in a rat model. Foot Ankle Int 2014;35(3):296; with permission.

SUMMARY

Improving the quality and strength of soft tissue repairs remains an important area of orthopedic research and innovation. The need for immobilization as well as early motion is an important, yet delicate, balance essential for the successful treatment of tendon repair and reconstruction. MSC-bearing sutures represent an emerging, and seemingly viable, biological augmentation to traditional suture repair. Two previous large studies using stem cell sutures in rat Achilles tendon models have demonstrated early increased biomechanical strength and significantly increased ultimate failure strength. The MSCs seem to remain locally at the repair site and enhance the histologic repair quality of the tendon collagen.

All of the currently available data in the literature are limited to basic science and animal models. Currently, Stem Cell Surgical, LLC is working through the regulatory pathway, which would support moving to clinical trials in the near future. Further studies, especially clinical studies, will be important to provide evidence about the safety and efficacy of MSC-bearing sutures.

REFERENCES

1. Aspenberg P. Stimulation of tendon repair: mechanical loading, GDFs and platelets. A mini-review. Int Orthop 2007;31:783–9.
2. Butler DL, Juncosa N, Dressler MR. Functional efficacy of tendon repair processes. Annu Rev Biomed Eng 2004;6:303–29.
3. Sharma P, Maffulli N. Tendon injury and tendinopathy: healing and repair. J Bone Joint Surg Am 2005;87:187–202.
4. Buckwalter JA. Effects of early motion on healing of musculoskeletal tissues. Hand Clin 1996;12:13–24.
5. Kellett J. Acute soft tissue injuries—a review of the literature. Med Sci Sports Exerc 1986;18:489–500.
6. Gelberman RH, Woo SL, Lothringer K, et al. Effects of early intermittent passive mobilization on healing canine flexor tendons. J Hand Surg 1982;7:170–5.
7. Gelberman RH, Boyer MI, Brodt MD, et al. The effect of gap formation at the repair site on the strength and excursion of intrasynovial flexor tendons: an experimental study on the early stages of tendon healing in dogs. J Bone Joint Surg Am 1999;81:975–82.
8. Mortensen NH, Saether J, Steinke MS, et al. Separation of tendon ends after Achilles tendon repair: a prospective, randomized, multicenter study. Orthopedics 1992;15:899–903.
9. Boyer MI, Goldfarb CA, Gelberman RH. Recent progress in flexor tendon healing. The modulation of tendon healing with rehabilitation variables. J Hand Ther 2005; 18(2):80–5.
10. Winters SC, Gelberman RH, Woo SL, et al. The effects of multiple strand suture methods on the strength and excursion of repaired intrasynovial flexor tendons: a biomechanical study in dogs. J Hand Surg 1998;23:97–104.
11. Caplan AI, Dennis JE. Mesenchymal stem cells as trophic mediators. J Cell Biochem 2006;98(5):1076–84.
12. Jones E, Yang X. Mesenchymal stem cells and bone regeneration: current status. Injury 2011;42:562–8.
13. Wang XJ, Dong Z, Zhong XH, et al. Transforming growth factor-beta1 enhanced vascular endothelial growth factor synthesis in mesenchymal stem cells. Biochem Biophys Res Commun 2008;365:548–54.

14. Young RG, Butler DL, Weber W, et al. Use of mesenchymal stem cells in a collagen matrix for Achilles tendon repair. J Orthop Res 1998;16:406–13.

15. Yao J, Korotkova T, Riboh J, et al. Bioactive sutures for tendon repair: assessment of a method of delivering pluripotential embryonic cells. J Hand Surg Am 2008; 33:1558–64.

16. Adams SB Jr, Thorpe MA, Parks BG, et al. Stem cell-bearing suture improves Achilles tendon healing in a rat model. Foot Ankle Int 2014;35(3):293–9.

17. Sutton MT, Fletcher D, Ghosh SK, et al. Antimicrobial properties of mesenchymal stem cells: therapeutic potential for cystic fibrosis infection, and treatment. Stem Cells Int 2016;2016:5303048.

18. Bagi Z, Kaley G. Where have all the stem cells gone? Circ Res 2009;104(3): 280–1.

19. Yao J, Woon CY, Behn A, et al. The effect of suture coated with mesenchymal stem cells and bioactive substrate on tendon repair strength in a rat model. J Hand Surg Am 2012;37:1639–45.

The Science Behind Wear Testing for Great Toe Implants for Hallux Rigidus

Judith F. Baumhauer, MD, MPH[a],*, Michele Marcolongo, PhD[b]

KEYWORDS

- Hydrogel • Toe implant • Hallux rigidus • PVA • Wear testing

KEY POINTS

- An orthopedic surgeon makes decisions about which implants to use to help his or her patients.
- Understanding the level of evidence supporting the use of the implant, and the rigor of the material testing, is critical to avoid repeating the failures resulting in bone loss and joint instability.
- The regulatory system allows for a 510K approval for implants as long as they can prove the new implant is "like" the old one in its use and application.
- Thus, no new knowledge is gained and the surgeon has no science to examine clinically, biomechanically, or histologically.

BACKGROUND

The function of articular cartilage is to provide a low-friction bearing surface enabling the joint to withstand weight bearing through the range of motion needed to perform activities of daily living. Various methods of repairing damaged articular cartilage surfaces have been proposed and a variety of implant materials have been tried in an attempt to decrease pain and improve function after cartilage repair. The majority of these techniques have significant limitations, including with loosening, malalignment/dislocation, implant fragmentation, and bone loss. A major cause of failure has been osteolysis and aseptic loosening owing to wear.[1]

The hydrogel made of polyvinyl alcohol and saline is a unique material used as an implant in the great toe for advanced stage arthritis. This material was developed to

Disclosure Statement: Dr J.F. Baumhauer is a paid consultant for Carticept Medical, DJ Orthopedics, Ferring Pharmaceuticals, Fidia Pharma USA Inc, Medtronic, Nextremity Solutions Inc, and Wright Medical Technology, Inc. Dr M. Marcolongo has nothing to disclose.
[a] Department of Orthopaedics, University of Rochester School of Medicine and Dentistry, Box 665 Elmwood Avenue, Rochester, NY 14642, USA; [b] Materials Science and Engineering, Drexel University, 3141 Chestnut Street, Philadelphia, PA 19014, USA
* Corresponding author.
E-mail address: Judy_Baumhauer@urmc.rochester.edu

1083-7515/16/© 2016 Elsevier Inc. All rights reserved.

mimic an artificial articular surface that has shock-absorbing ability, high wear resistance, and wear particulate biocompatibility, properties necessary for suitability as a biomaterial intended to replace damaged cartilage. Prior implants made of silicone were used for great toe arthritis and failed owing to poor wear characteristics. Understanding the differences between the various materials and the biomechanical testing performed on these materials allows the surgeon to make educated selection on implants to use in the treatment of their patients.

REGULATORY PATHWAY

The Food and Drug Administration (FDA) regulates medical devices in the United States with different levels of regulatory oversight depending on the classification of the device. The 2 most common regulator pathways are the 510(k) premarket submission and the more rigorous premarket approval (PMA).

The FDA evaluates medical devices including arthroplasty products by 2 main pathways, premarket notification or 510(k) PMA. The former requires demonstration that the device is substantially equivalent to a predicate device. Submitted data typically involve laboratory testing demonstrating that the new device introduces no new safety risks. Any devices not substantially equivalent to existing products follow the more stringent PMA pathway, requiring evidence of device safety and effectiveness. For a PMA application, clinical data from a large randomized clinical study is required to demonstrate safety and effectiveness, in addition to comprehensive laboratory studies characterizing the device properties, functionality, and safety.

The majority of total joint replacement and hemiarthroplasty implants (using materials already widely used such as titanium, ceramic, polyethylene, and silicone) reach market via a 510(k) submission that, depending on availability of predicate device data, may or may not include wear testing simulating indication-specific in vivo conditions and animal implantation of wear particulate.

Because this was the first use of a polyvinyl alcohol hydrogel material for cartilage repair, the FDA required the PMA pathway for this polyvinyl alcohol polymer (PVA) implant, the most stringent type of device marketing application required by the FDA. In addition to the PMA requirement for large randomized clinical studies to prove safety and effectiveness of the device, a PMA requires extensive testing of the material's suitability as a cartilage replacement material.

OTHER HEMIARTHROPLASTY MATERIAL CONCERNS

Hemiarthroplasty initially began with implants into the proximal phalanx, and have evolved to include 1 implant for the metatarsal head side of the joint. These implants are designed to resurface the first metatarsophalangeal (MTP) joint while maintaining or preserving motion.[2]

Although some of these implants have been available for more than 50 years, few studies have been published investigating the effectiveness of these implants. In addition, material concerns exist with silicone implants, as reported in the literature. Unlike hydrogels, silicone elastomers are nonbiphasic, hydrophobic, and not well-lubricated in the body.

Silicone orthopedic prostheses introduced in the early 1960s were initially believed to be durable and biocompatible with good initial clinical results. Occurrence of inflammatory responses is now well-recognized with these types of implants and is attributed to foreign body giant cell reaction to silicone particles.[3–5] Although the implant itself is inert, abrasion and fatigue fracture of the implants was found to produce microscopic particles that caused inflammatory synovitis, a complication not readily identifiable without laboratory wear testing modeling physiologic load and articulation conditions as well as wear debris animal testing (**Fig. 1**). Complications secondary to the silicone microfragmentation include periimplant bone resorption, subchondral cyst formation, deformity, and silicone lymphadenopathy.[6,7] The addition of silica (silicon dioxide) during the manufacture of silicone prostheses has also been identified as a potential material source known to induce inflammation and fibrosis. Wear may increase exposure to silica and may contribute to the cellular response.[8]

Overall, from an engineering perspective, the 2 most relevant complications are device breakage and device wear. Specifically, the previously studied double-stemmed, hinged prosthesis spans both sides of the joint and is designed to allow the toe to continue to bend after implantation. This subjects the device to repetitive bending moments that cause device fracture at either the stems or at the hinge, which is a stress concentrator. The hinged silicone prosthesis was initially believed to be durable and biocompatible. During the early 1980s, however, reports of premature wear and silicone synovitis began to appear in the literature.[3] Although the implant itself is inert, abrasion of the implants was found to produce microscopic particles that caused an inflammatory synovitis. Implant wear was also found to cause a silicone particulate lymphadenitis and cystic osteolysis in cancellous bone adjacent to the implants.

POLYVINYL ALCOHOL POLYMER HYDROGEL IMPLANT

The synthetic implant (Cartiva Synthetic Cartilage Implant [SCI]; Cartiva, Inc, Alpharetta, GA) is a hydrogel polymer with properties similar to those of cartilage. The material is composed of 2 components, a water-soluble synthetic PVA and normal saline, which is formulated and device geometry fixed through a thermal-physical mixture. This PVA material structure mimics key properties of load-bearing cartilage: permeability, shock absorption, and lubrication. During loading, fluid migration provides impact load damping and self-lubrication, reducing friction.[9]

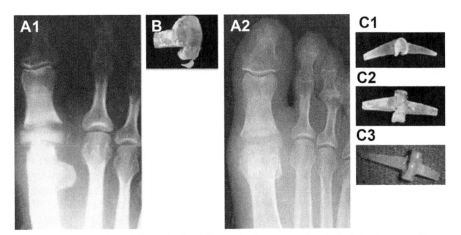

Fig. 1. Silicone implant failure. (*A1*) Radiograph demonstrating failed single-stem silicone arthroplasty. (*B*) Failed silicone hemiarthroplasty implant. (*A2*) Radiograph demonstrating placement of double-stem silicone implant. (*C1–C3*) Examples of failures of double-stem implants. (*From* Hirose CB, Coughlin MJ, Stevens FR. Arthritis of the Foot and Ankle. Chapter 19. In: Coughlin MJ, Saltzman CL, Anderson RB, et al, editors. Mann's surgery of the foot and ankle, vol. 1. 9th edition. Philadelphia: Elsevier Saunders; 2013. p. 982, 985; with permission.)

Polyvinyl Alcohol Polymer Hydrogel Preclinical Testing

Testing requirements include a broad range of studies to demonstrate the suitability of the material for its intended purpose, including biocompatibility, material properties testing, functional and fatigue testing, chemical characterization, animal testing, and extensive wear and in vivo wear particulate testing (**Table 1**). Biocompatibility testing conducted in the implant and instrumentation using ISO 10993 demonstrated the materials are biocompatible for the intended use and do not illicit a biologic reaction. Material testing included the evaluation of various properties such as confined compression (aggregate modulus), unconfined compression, creep, shear, hydration properties, and cyclic stress against the logarithmic of cycles to failure (S-N). These material testing properties, including load to failure were compared with similar values reported in the literature for articular cartilage, demonstrating that the PVA hydrogel implant wear characteristics were suitable for use in the first MTP joint.

Mechanical fatigue and wear testing were carried out using the anticipated clinical loading as calculated through joint and gait modeling based on published literature. The fatigue and wear testing demonstrated the device can withstand a simulated 5 years of continual cyclic loading in excess of clinically relevant loading values, as well as withstand simulated 5 year of articulating wear. All benchtop testing values are indicative that the PVA hydrogel device is designed to withstand the physiologic conditions of the first MTP joint.

Pushout testing was conducted to quantify the fixation of PVA hydrogel devices implanted into model tissue/bone constructs using the PVA hydrogel instrumentation and the procedure that will be specified in the PMA product's instructions for use and demonstrated the implantation could easily be achieved and the implants were secure in the cavity.

Results of the 1-year goat implant study demonstrated that the study objectives were met in that there was no local or systemic toxicity, no inflammatory reaction around the implant, and osteolytic bone loss. In comparison with controls (empty defect), there were nonsignificant changes to the opposing tibial surface and no difference in the occurrence of the presence of subarticular cysts. No device dislodgment was observed. There was no instance of device fragmentation and the device was retained in all instances.

Polyvinyl Alcohol Polymer Hydrogel Wear and Particulate Testing

Wear testing methodology

Because the PVA hydrogel implant involved a new material used in an orthopedic implant, there was considerable focus and attention to ensure that this material would be suitable for use in the MTP joint. This testing required the development of a new wear testing fixture and testing methodology to simulate the wear environment of the first MTP joint. Simulated wear under conditions more challenging than in the human first MTP joint was critical to demonstrate the long-term durability of the PVA hydrogel device and to quantify the wear particles. The wear environment simulated a normal gait cycle and peak loading experienced during walking (**Figs. 2 and 3**).

To achieve this wear environment in vitro, a 6-station wear simulator was developed for MTP joint articulation to provide the degrees, loading, and controls necessary to apply 5,000,000 cycles of a walking gait to multiple PVA hydrogel devices simultaneously. The PVA hydrogel devices were articulated against opposing wear surfaces (cartilage) that would most accurately simulate the environment of the first MTP joint (**Fig. 4**).

Table 1
Preclinical testing summary

Extensive Preclinical Testing Components		
Biocompatibility	Cytotoxicity L929 MEM elution Cytotoxicity direct Sensitization Kligman maximization Irritation/intracutaneous IC injection Acute systemic toxicity systemic injection test Subchronic toxicity medial femoral condyle implantation study Chronic toxicity medial femoral condyle implantation study Genotoxicity Ames reverse mutation Genotoxicity chromosomal aberration assay Genotoxicity rodent bone marrow micronucleus assay Implantation bone implantation in femoral condyle Pyrogenicity	

Material properties	Unconfined compression
	    Loading of unconfined devices to achieve 10%, 20%, 30% and 40% strain to measure deformation resistance of the matrix and determine compatibility of the device with surrounding native tissue
	Confined compression
	    Devices confined in compression fixture with 5%, 10%, 15%, 20%, and 25% strain applied to assess matrix stiffness at equilibrium (ie, when load-induced fluid flow has ceased)
	Shear
	    Devices seated between test blocks that are moved apart perpendicularly until failure; thereby, providing a baseline understanding of the simple shear properties of the material
	Compressive creep
	    Simulated use loading in confined compression fixture to elucidate structural changes because equilibrium swelling properties are sensitive to the nature and stability of the hydrogel cross-links
	Hydration properties
	    Devices dehydrated at ambient conditions followed by rehydration
	S-N analysis
	    Devices loaded in a confined fixture to 8, 12, 18, and 24 MPa out to 5,000,000 cycles	

Functional testing - fatigue		Cycles – 5 million Test surface – finished PVA hydrogel device vs stainless steel Simulated axial load – 4 MPa
Chemical characterization	Testing of PVA resin, nonsterile and sterile devices, as well as sterile devices after compressive fatigue cycling for characterization	Differential scanning calorimetry Fourier transform infrared spectroscopy Gel permeation chromatography Nuclear MR Infrared analysis Physicochemical analysis X-ray diffraction Density and specific gravity Exhaustive extraction High-pressure liquid chromatography

(continued on next page)

Table 1 *(continued)*		
Animal studies	1 y goat – implant in stifle of 8 mature goats; control defect in 4 goats	High field strength MRI system for morphology and quantitative T2 and T1-rho parameters Histologic processing Biomechanical testing
Wear testing	Articulation of PVA Hydrogel (Cartiva SCI) device vs cartilage to assess the propensity for wear	Cycles – 5 Million Test surface – finished PVA hydrogel (Cartiva SCI) device vs cartilage Simulated axial load – 4 MPa Particulate analysis – SEM low angle light scattering
Wear debris/ particulate implant	6 mo particulate implant study in 16 rabbits	Particulate injection in rabbit knee - particulate from 5 million wear cycles replicated and injected via bolus in quantity 9× that generated during testing 3 and 6 mo – histology and pathology per ISO standards show no bioreactivity

Abbreviations: IC, intracutaneus; ISO, International Organization for Standardization; PVA, polyvinyl alcohol polymer; SEM, scanning electron microscopy.

Each cartilage opposing surface was constructed of fresh cartilage excised from the joint and dissected to accommodate the wear testing simulator and sliding distance required (**Fig. 5**). The cartilage sample was held within a stainless steel test fixture (**Fig. 6**) for articulation against the PVA hydrogel implant device. Each of the 6 PVA hydrogel implant test articles were housed in a separate test station in the wear simulator and maintained in phosphate-buffered saline at $37 \pm 3°C$. The individual test station setup is depicted in **Fig. 7**.

Polyvinyl Alcohol Polymer Hydrogel Implant Wear Results

The PVA hydrogel devices demonstrated only minor wear during the 5,000,000 cycles of testing. This total number of cycles represents a wear scenario spanning 5 years under worst case wear conditions. The PVA hydrogel devices were tested under

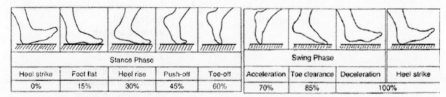

Fig. 2. Stages of normal gait. Various stages of normal walking gait. (*From* Sammarco GJ, Hockenbury RT. Biomechanics of the foot and ankle. Chapter 9. In: Nordin M, et al, editor. Basic biomechanics of the musculoskeletal system. 4th edition. Philadelphia: Lippincott Williams & Wilkins; 2012. p. 227; with permission.)

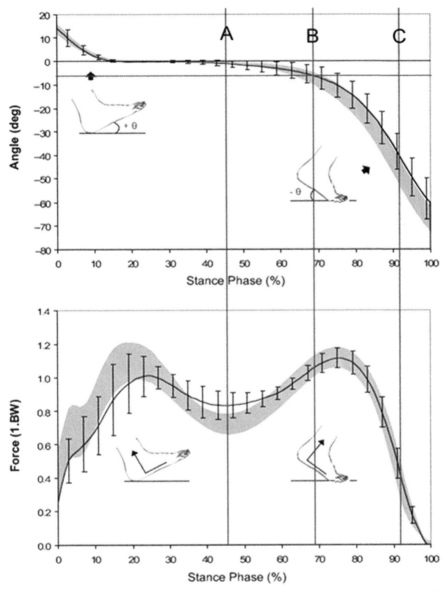

Fig. 3. Motion and loading of the foot during walking. The gray area represents the average motion and loading for normal patients and the solid line represents patients with rheumatoid arthritis. The top graph measures foot angle, where negative values can be attributed primarily to motion of the metatarsophalangeal (MTP) joint. The bottom graph shows the contact force, which includes both heel and forefoot forces. Line A in the graph corresponds with heel rise stage of walking, when contact forces are primarily concentrated in the forefoot. This corresponds with around 350 ms in **Fig. 2**, when the first MTP begins to experience significant load. Line B correlates with the push-off phase of walking, which occurs about halfway between heel rise and toe-off. This correlates with around 475 ms in B. Although significant loads are experienced between lines A and B, only minimal motion occurs. Therefore, this portion of the load profile is not expected to contribute to wear significantly. Line C corresponds with a time shortly before toe-off,

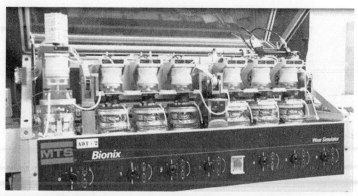

Fig. 4. Six station wear simulator during polyvinyl alcohol polymer hydrogel (Cartiva SCI) testing. (*Courtesy of* Cartiva (TM), Alpharetta, GA; with permission.)

maximum loads throughout the entire walking cycle without interruption of loading, in excess of what is observed physiologically.

Polyvinyl Alcohol Polymer Hydrogel Wear Debris

The wear debris particulate collected during the PVA hydrogel implant wear study was analyzed for size, total quantity and particle morphology using both laser light scattering and scanning electron microscopy technology. The particles were round to oval or elongated in shape with an average aspect ratio of 1.7, but not excessively so and thus do not classify as fibers. The average particle equivalent circle diameter was 3.8 microns.

The average total mass of debris collected per device over 5 million cycles was 0.18% of the initial mass of the test articles, well below the acceptance criteria of 100 mg over 5 million cycles. The volumetric wear rate was determined to be 1.50 mm^3 per year. This is considerably lower than the threshold wear rate to induce osteolysis for ultra-high molecular weight polyethylene (UHMWPE), which is 80 mm^3 per year (or a linear penetration rate of 0.1 mm/y).[10] Not only is the wear rate of the PVA hydrogel implant lower than that of UHMWPE, UHMWPE particulate cause intense inflammation as compared with PVA hydrogels.[9]

To assess the biocompatibility of PVA hydrogel wear debris, particulate was generated for intraarticular implantation in the New Zealand white rabbit model. Particulate characteristics affecting the in vivo biological response—particle size, morphology, and total amount of debris—were consistent with those of the debris generated during the wear study. The particulate was injected into the rabbit knees, a joint 6.5 times

---

when the MTP is quickly rotating, but is not being significantly loaded. This corresponds with 600 ms in **Fig. 2**. Owing to the low load, motion occurring after 600 ms is also not expected to significantly contribute to wear. Therefore, there is essentially a window of around 125 ms, from push-off to toe-off, where the combination of motion and loading are expected to account for the vast majority of wear. The x axis of this figure measures stance phase, which accounts for only 60% of a 1000 ms complete gait that includes both stance and swing phases. (*Adapted from* Turner DE, Helliwell PS, Emery P, et al. The impact of rheumatoid arthritis on foot function in the early stages of disease: a clinical case series. BMC Musculoskelet Disord 2006;7:102; with permission.)

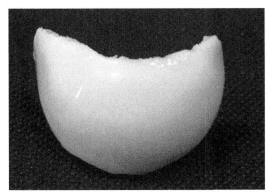

Fig. 5. Cartilage specimen used for wear testing.

smaller than the human first MTP joint as determined via synovial fluid volume comparison.[11,12] The total mass per sample injected into each rabbit knee was 3.9 mg, a safety factor of approximately 9-fold the maximum mass of wear debris.

The animals were assessed via histologic tissue processing and pathology per ISO 10993-6 tests for local effects after implantation at 3 and 6 months. Both time interval testing noted no complications. All animals survived to the scheduled 3-month and 6-month termination time points. There were no test article-related adverse changes in viabilities, physical examinations, clinical observations, administration site scores, body weight, and gross or systemic pathology of animals assigned at the 3-month and 6-month intervals. Histomorphometry evaluations performed on RAM-11 stained knee joint sections indicated that intraarticular injection of PVA hydrogel implant particulate did not elicit a significantly greater local reaction compared with the sodium chloride control treatment at either time point. There was a reduction in macrophage activity for both treated and control animals at the 6-month interval, but the differences were not significant. Histopathology showed no microscopic changes related to the test article and no variations in scores were significant. There were no treatment-related changes in the morphology or integrity of the cartilage surfaces, synovium,

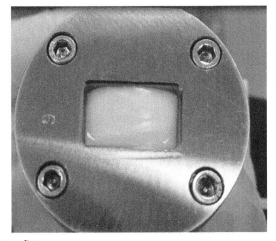

Fig. 6. Cartilage test fixture.

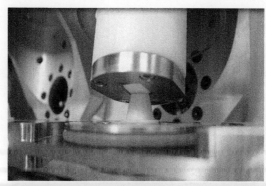

Fig. 7. Polyvinyl alcohol polymer hydrogel (Cartiva SCI) (bottom) versus cartilage (*top*) test station. (*Courtesy of* Cartiva (TM), Alpharetta, GA; with permission.)

joint capsule, or underlying bone. Treatment with the test article produced no evidence of arthritis at 3 or 6 months and there was no evidence of systemic toxicity. The test article was found to be a nonirritant in this model.

Overall, the PVA hydrogel device demonstrated wear resistance under worst conditions of testing and provided an overall wear rate significantly lower than that published to induce osteolysis for UHMWPE devices.

In Vivo Clinical Wear Findings

The safety and effectiveness of PVA hydrogel implant (Cartiva SCI) was evaluated in prospective randomized trial, MOTION Study in 236 subjects comparing the PVA hydrogel implant to fusion. The study demonstrated that the PVA hydrogel implant provided significant reduction in pain, improvement in function and subject's range of motion. The results were demonstrated to be equivalent to fusion, the standard

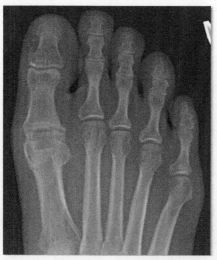
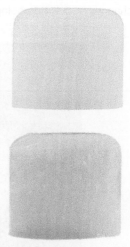

Fig. 8. 1 Year MOTION study explant. Radiograph at 1 year, before explant. Cartiva SCI implant before use (*right top*) and explanted at 1 year with no signs of wear, degradation or material loss (*right bottom*). (*Courtesy of* Cartiva (TM), Alpharetta, GA; with permission.)

of care.[13] In the MOTION study, a small group of subjects required removal of the PVA hydrogel device for persistent pain (9.2%), which was comparable with the subjects requiring revision or hardware removal in the fusion group (12%). The devices removed from MOTION study patients were examined and did not demonstrate wear or damage. There were no device removals for device fracture, fragmentation, infection or inflammatory reaction (**Fig. 8**).

SUMMARY

An orthopedic surgeon makes decisions about which implants to use to help his or her patients. Understanding not only the level of clinical evidence supporting the use of the implant, but also the rigor of the material testing both mechanical and histologic, is critical to avoid repeating the failures resulting in bone loss and joint instability, such as that seen with silicone within the foot and ankle. The regulatory system allows for a 510(k) approval for implants as long as they can prove the new implant is "like" the old one in its use and application and therefore no new knowledge is gained and the surgeon has no science to examine clinically, biomechanically or histological-ly. This PVA hydrogel implant (Cartiva SCI) has provided scientific evidence of clinical effectiveness in a prior study and provides a great example of robust biomechanical and histologic testing for the surgeon to share with his or her patient when considering its use.

REFERENCES

1. Baker MI, Walsh SP, Schwartz Z, et al. A review of polyvinyl alcohol and its uses in cartilage and orthopedic applications. J Biomed Mater Res B Appl Biomater 2012;100(5):1451–7.
2. Giza E, Sullivan MR. First metatarsophalangeal hemiarthroplasty for grade III and IV hallux rigidus. Tech Foot Ankle Surg 2005;4(1):10–7.
3. Lemon RA, Engber WD, McBeath AA. A complication of silastic hemiarthroplasty in bunion surgery. Foot Ankle 1984;4(5):262–6.
4. Gordon M, Bullough PG. Synovial and osseous inflammation in failed silicone-rubber prostheses. J Bone Joint Surg Am 1982;64(4):574–80.
5. Lanzetta M, Herbert TJ, Conolly WB. Silicone synovitis. A perspective. J Hand Surg Br 1994;19(4):479–84.
6. Naidu SH, Beredjiklian P, Adler L, et al. In vivo inflammatory response to silicone elastomer particulate debris. J Hand Surg Am 1996;21(3):496–500.
7. Sammarco GJ, Tabatowski K. Silicone lymphadenopathy associated with failed prosthesis of the hallux: a case report and literature review. Foot Ankle 1992; 13(5):273–6.
8. Kusaka T, Nakayama M, Nakamura K, et al. Effect of silica particle size on macro-phage inflammatory responses. PLoS One 2014;9(3):e92634.
9. Oka M, Ushio K, Kumar P, et al. Development of artificial articular cartilage. Proc Inst Mech Eng H 2000;214(1):59–68.
10. Jacobs CA, Christensen CP, Greenwald AS, et al. Clinical performance of highly cross-linked polyethylenes in total hip arthroplasty. J Bone Joint Surg Am 2007; 89(12):2779–86.
11. Knox P, Levick R, McDonald JN. Synovial fluid – its mass, macromolecular con-tent and pressure in major limb joints of the rabbit. Q J Exp Physiol 1988;73: 33–45.

12. Kingston A, Tomas A, Ghosh-Ray S, et al. Does running cause metatarsophalangeal joint effusions? A comparison of synovial fluid volumes on MRI in athletes before and after running. Skeletal Radiol 2009;38:499–504.

13. Baumhauer JB, Singh D, Glazebrook M, et al. Prospective, randomized, multi-centered clinical trial assessing safety and efficacy of a synthetic cartilage implant versus first metatarsophalangeal arthrodesis in advanced hallux rigidus. Foot Ankle Int 2016;37(5):457–69.

The Science Behind Surgical Innovations of the Forefoot

Judith F. Baumhauer, MD, MPH[a],*, Michele Marcolongo, PhD[b]

KEYWORDS

- Orthopaedic devices • Forefoot • Surgical techniques

KEY POINTS

- Forefoot surgery has gone through a lot of innovation over the last 5 years.
- Surgeons have the obligation to select the procedures and implants that are going to lead to the best outcomes for patients.
- By understanding the science behind each implant, and the advantages and disadvantages of these technologies, the proper selection of appropriate devices can be made to obtain the best possible results for patients.

BACKGROUND

The area of foot and ankle surgery has made tremendous advances in the last 10 years. The global foot and ankle device market forecast for 2015 to 2020 is expected to reach nearly 5.5 billion dollars resulting in an increase of 7.2%. As orthopedic surgeons, we should be selective in directing the use of orthopedic devices to improve the care we provide for our patients. It is critical that we look at these new devices that come to market with scientific rigor. It is also important that we continue to advance innovation yet study it appropriately, as this will help us as orthopedic surgeons to support our primary objective of providing cost-effective care.

One of the areas of foot and ankle surgery that has had particular attention over the last 5 years has been forefoot surgery. Common procedures include correction of the lessor metatarsophalangeal joints and hammertoe deformities, specifically metatarsal shortening osteotomies and proximal interphalangeal joint fusions. The goals of these

Disclosure Statement: Dr J.F. Baumhauer is a paid consultant for Carticept Medical, DJ Orthopaedics, Ferring Pharmaceuticals, Fidia Pharma USA Inc, Medtronic, Nextremity Solutions Inc, and Wright Medical Technology, Inc; Dr M. Marcolongo has nothing to disclose.
[a] Department of Orthopaedics, University of Rochester School of Medicine and Dentistry, Box 665 Elmwood Avenue, Rochester, NY 14642, USA; [b] Department of Materials Science and Engineering, Materials Science and Engineering, Drexel University, 3141 Chestnut Street, Philadelphia, PA 19014, USA
* Corresponding author.
E-mail address: Judy_Baumhauer@urmc.rochester.edu

surgeries are to improve patient function and allow patients to fit into shoes more comfortably.

METATARSAL SHORTENING OSTEOTOMIES

Varieties of techniques exist for metatarsal shortening osteotomies and they have been plagued with complications and unreliable outcomes. Goals of this surgery are to decrease the length of the metatarsal, to decrease the lever arm and tension of the adjacent soft tissue structures, and allow for improved alignment and soft tissue balancing of the metatarsophalangeal joint. With these goals comes the need to accurately measure the amount of shortening as well as maintain the bone alignment in that new position without malunion, nonunion, displacement, or rotational deformity. The upper extremity surgeons have performed shortening osteotomies of the ulna for impingement or malalignment for years. Using a plate with a saw cut capture, this ulnar shortening osteotomy has been a reliable operation to allow controlled shortening and compression and avoid any malalignment. Translating that successful operation to the weight-bearing zone of the foot, specifically the metatarsal, required some additional scientific proof that the device could withstand weight-bearing forces without hardware complications. Recent publications have demonstrated the difficulty in using traditional simple plates and screws for the foot without any specific design for this metatarsal shortening operation.[1] These challenges resulted in hardware breakage and nonunion of the osteotomy. It is important for orthopedic surgeons to understand the science behind the devices to appropriately select the correct implants and instrumentation for the operation.

Fig. 1A demonstrates the metatarsal shortening plate with a saw cut capture mimicking the ulnar shortening procedure. It allows up to 6 mm of shortening of the metatarsal through an oblong screw hole. There are also locking screws distally to add additional stability. The plate itself has a keel to provide rotational stability and alignment. **Fig. 1**B demonstrates the static 4-point bending stiffness for a single-plane plate traditionally used for a diaphyseal ulnar shortening osteotomy and the multiplane plate. The multiplane plate is 4 times as stiff as demonstrated on this normalized graph.

DeSandis and colleagues[1] published on the delayed unions occurring from diaphyseal osteotomies that were transverse and stabilized with a single-plane dorsal plate. The incidence of delayed union of the osteotomies was stated at 75.8% representing

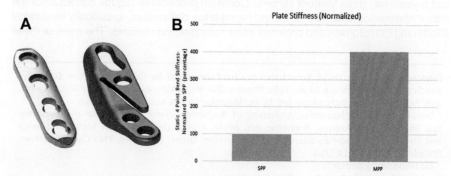

Fig. 1. (*A*) Metatarsal shortening plate with a saw cut capture mimicking the ulnar shortening procedure. (*B*) Graph depicting the static 4-point bending stiffness for a single-plane plate traditionally used for a diaphyseal ulnar shortening osteotomy and the multiplane plate. (*Courtesy of* Nextremity Solutions, Inc, Warsaw, Indiana; with permission.)

69 of 91 osteotomies. Six out of 69 delayed unions were considered nonunions at 1 year, representing a 6.6% nonunion rate. Galluch and colleagues[2] published on 126 diaphyseal osteotomies of the lesser metatarsals with a retrospective review looking for osteotomy union, symptomatic relief, and complications associated with the procedure. The average time of follow-up was 8.8 months. The fixation was described as a single-plane dorsal plate. Their complications included 5 patients with transfer lesions and one patient who developed a nonunion. Overall their rate of union was 99.2%. The postoperative course consisted of non–weight bearing for the first 2 weeks and protected weight bearing after that time frame and weight bearing to tolerance at 2 months. With the added stability of the multiplanar plate, weight bearing can begin as soon as 1 week postoperatively with the initial week essentially to allow for wound healing and the avoidance of excessive swelling.[2]

With the single-plane plate, there is no ability to dial in the amount of shortening. The amount of shortening is dictated by the transverse resection of bone. Another common osteotomy is the Weil osteotomy to allow for metatarsal shortening through the metaphyseal portion of the neck of the metatarsal. There have been multiple complications described with a Weil osteotomy, the most common is coined *the floating toe* because of the persistent imbalance of intrinsic tendons and plantar translation of the metatarsal head. The Weil osteotomy is commonly secured with a single screw. Highlander and colleagues[3] published a literature review examining the outcomes of the Weil osteotomy. They found 17 articles that qualified for analysis, resulting in 1131 Weil osteotomies. The most commonly reported complication of a Weil osteotomy was a floating toe reported in 233 cases and an overall occurrence of 36%. There was a recurrence of the original toe deformity of 15%. Transverse metatarsalgia was reported in 7% of the cases; delayed union, nonunion, and malunion were reported in 3% of cases.[3] Like the diaphyseal osteotomies that are performed transversely, *a difficulty exists* in assessing the degree of shortening that is performed intraoperatively with a Weil osteotomy.

One factor that will increase osteotomy healing is the fusion surface area. **Fig. 2** displays the contact surface area in millimeters for transverse, Weil, and oblique osteotomies. With the oblique osteotomy, the surface area available for healing is significantly increased.

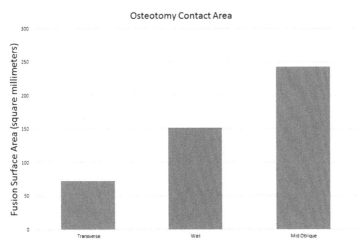

Osteotomy Contact Area

Fig. 2. Contact surface area in millimeters for transverse, Weil, and oblique osteotomies. (*Courtesy of* Nextremity Solutions, Inc, Warsaw, Indiana; with permission.)

The multiplanar plate structure, the oblique osteotomy saw capture incorporation within the plate, and the ability to stabilize the osteotomy with locking screws and select the amount of shortening that is required are all the advantages to the advancement of the new plate construct. It is through these scientific advancements that our patients will benefit.

Another component of a hammertoe deformity is a proximal interphalangeal joint flexion contracture. This flexion contracture can cause rubbing in the shoe and pain and, when severe, even open wounds due to the abrasion from the shoe and subsequent infection. Traditional treatment of these fixed flexion contractures is a resection of the distal portion of the proximal phalanx and the proximal portion of the middle phalanx and fusion of those two surfaces. Implants to date have consisted of Kirschner wire fixation, which traditionally requires removal at 4 to 6 weeks to avoid ongoing infection, intramedullary screw fixation, and memory metal-type implants. Like any form of fusion, compression and rigid fixation are critical to allow direct bone contact and intramembranous bone healing. The implants to date have not demonstrated compression to occur across the proximal interphalangeal joint surfaces. Rather than being a compression device, the implants have been a static stabilizing device. Complications with a static device include the potential for implant failure by breakage or dislodgement.

Recognizing the need for compression, an implant has been designed to allow for compression through the use of nitinol anchor implants into the proximal and middle phalanx and a deployment of a rigid polyetheretherketone (PEEK) cylindrical tube and pulley system allowing for apposition of the two bone surfaces. To assess the degree of compression and maintenance of compression over a 12-week period of time, the

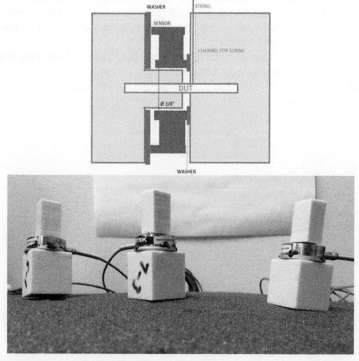

Fig. 3. Hammertoe test device (ProxiFuse). DUT, device under test. (*Courtesy of* Cartiva, Alpharetta, Georgia; with permission.)

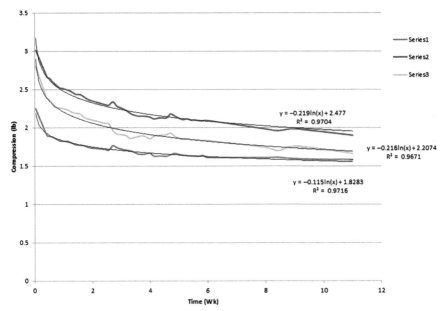

$$y = -0.219\ln(x) + 2.477$$
$$R^2 = 0.9704$$

$$y = -0.216\ln(x) + 2.2074$$
$$R^2 = 0.9671$$

$$y = -0.115\ln(x) + 1.8283$$
$$R^2 = 0.9716$$

Fig. 4. ProxiFuse compression over 12 week recovery period. (*Courtesy of Cartiva, Alpharetta, Georgia; with permission.*)

hammertoe test device (ProxiFuse, Cartiva, Inc, Alpharetta, GA) was implanted into simulated bone material with a standard technique and placed in a foam mat to dampen the effects of vibration (**Fig. 3**). Initial force readings were taken immediately and at 8 hours. The implanted devices were monitored daily with the compression force recorded for the first 6 weeks of the test. During weeks 7 through 12, compression readings were obtained weekly. The graphic representation of the data over the 12-week test period is shown in **Fig. 4**. The mean starting force was 5.1 lb with a range from 4.8 to 5.5 lb. The ending force mean was 1.72 lb with a range of 1.6 to 1.9 lb. Based on these compression data, the hammertoe device produced significant initial compression; although the compression force did decline during the study period, there was still a compressive load that represented 34% of the original force at 12 weeks. Another advantage of this implant is that the PEEK cylindrical tube is radiolucent, which allows for excellent visibility of the opposing bone surfaces for interpretation of bony bridging.

SUMMARY

As surgeons, we have the ability to select the appropriate procedures and implants that are going to lead to the best outcomes for our patients. Understanding the science behind each implant and the advantages and disadvantages of these technologies will guide us into the selection of appropriate devices to obtain the best possible functional results for our patients.

REFERENCES

1. DeSandis B, Ellis SJ, Levitsky M, et al. Rate of union after segmental midshaft shortening osteotomy of the lesser metatarsals. Foot Ankle Int 2015;36(10): 1190–5.

2. Galluch DB, Bohay DR, Anderson JG. Midshaft metatarsal segmental osteotomy with open reduction and internal fixation. Foot Ankle Int 2007;28(2):169–74.

3. Highlander P, VonHerbulis E, Gonzalez A, et al. Complications of the Weil osteotomy. Foot Ankle Spec 2011;4(3):165–70.

Index

Note: Page numbers of article titles are in **boldface** type.

Foot Ankle Clin N Am 21 (2016) 909–939
http://dx.doi.org/10.1016/S1083-7515(16)30106-1
1083-7515/16

foot.theclinics.com

UNITED STATES POSTAL SERVICE®
Statement of Ownership, Management, and Circulation
(All Periodicals Publications Except Requester Publications)

1. Publication Title	2. Publication Number	3. Filing Date
FOOT AND ANKLE CLINICS OF NORTH AMERICA	016 – 368	9/18/2016

4. Issue Frequency	5. Number of Issues Published Annually	6. Annual Subscription Price
MAR, JUN, SEP, DEC	4	$299.00

7. Complete Mailing Address of Known Office of Publication (Not printer) (Street, city, county, state, and ZIP+4®)

ELSEVIER INC.
360 PARK AVENUE SOUTH
NEW YORK, NY 10010-1710

Contact Person: STEPHEN R. BUSHING
Telephone (include area code): 215-239-3688

8. Complete Mailing Address of Headquarters or General Business Office of Publisher (Not printer)

ELSEVIER INC.
360 PARK AVENUE SOUTH
NEW YORK, NY 10010-1710

9. Full Names and Complete Mailing Addresses of Publisher, Editor, and Managing Editor (Do not leave blank)

Publisher (Name and complete mailing address)

ADRIANNE BRIGIDO, ELSEVIER INC.
1600 JOHN F KENNEDY BLVD. SUITE 1800
PHILADELPHIA, PA 19103-2899

Editor (Name and complete mailing address)

LAUREN BOYLE, ELSEVIER INC.
1600 JOHN F KENNEDY BLVD. SUITE 1800
PHILADELPHIA, PA 19103-2899

Managing Editor (Name and complete mailing address)

PATRICK MANLEY, ELSEVIER INC.
1600 JOHN F KENNEDY BLVD. SUITE 1800
PHILADELPHIA, PA 19103-2899

10. Owner (Do not leave blank. If the publication is owned by a corporation, give the name and address of the corporation immediately followed by the names and addresses of all stockholders owning or holding 1 percent or more of the total amount of stock. If not owned by a corporation, give the names and addresses of the individual owners. If owned by a partnership or other unincorporated firm, give its name and address as well as those of each individual owner. If the publication is published by a nonprofit organization, give its name and address.)

Full Name	Complete Mailing Address
WHOLLY OWNED SUBSIDIARY OF REED/ELSEVIER, US HOLDINGS	1600 JOHN F KENNEDY BLVD. SUITE 1800 PHILADELPHIA, PA 19103-2899

11. Known Bondholders, Mortgagees, and Other Security Holders Owning or Holding 1 Percent or More of Total Amount of Bonds, Mortgages, or Other Securities. If none, check box ▶ ☐ None

Full Name	Complete Mailing Address
N/A	

12. Tax Status (For completion by nonprofit organizations authorized to mail at nonprofit rates) (Check one)
The purpose, function, and nonprofit status of this organization and the exempt status for federal income tax purposes:
☐ Has Not Changed During Preceding 12 Months
☐ Has Changed During Preceding 12 Months (Publisher must submit explanation of change with this statement)

13. Publication Title	14. Issue Date for Circulation Data Below
FOOT AND ANKLE CLINICS OF NORTH AMERICA	JUNE 2016

15. Extent and Nature of Circulation		Average No. Copies Each Issue During Preceding 12 Months	No. Copies of Single Issue Published Nearest to Filing Date
a. Total Number of Copies (Net press run)		470	482
b. Paid Circulation (By Mail and Outside the Mail)	(1) Mailed Outside-County Paid Subscriptions Stated on PS Form 3541 (Include paid distribution above nominal rate, advertiser's proof copies, and exchange copies)	257	285
	(2) Mailed In-County Paid Subscriptions Stated on PS Form 3541 (Include paid distribution above nominal rate, advertiser's proof copies, and exchange copies)	0	0
	(3) Paid Distribution Outside the Mails Including Sales Through Dealers and Carriers, Street Vendors, Counter Sales, and Other Paid Distribution Outside USPS®	91	119
	(4) Paid Distribution by Other Classes of Mail Through the USPS (e.g., First-Class Mail®)	0	0
c. Total Paid Distribution (Sum of 15b (1), (2), (3), and (4))	▶	348	404
d. Free or Nominal Rate Distribution (By Mail and Outside the Mail)	(1) Free or Nominal Rate Outside-County Copies included on PS Form 3541	19	48
	(2) Free or Nominal Rate In-County Copies Included on PS Form 3541	0	0
	(3) Free or Nominal Rate Copies Mailed at Other Classes Through the USPS (e.g., First-Class Mail)	0	0
	(4) Free or Nominal Rate Distribution Outside the Mail (Carriers or other means)	0	0
e. Total Free or Nominal Rate Distribution (Sum of 15d (1), (2), (3) and (4))	▶	19	48
f. Total Distribution (Sum of 15c and 15e)	▶	367	452
g. Copies not Distributed (See Instructions to Publishers #4 (page #3))	▶	103	30
h. Total (Sum of 15f and g)	▶	470	482
i. Percent Paid (15c divided by 15f times 100)		95%	89%

* If you are claiming electronic copies, go to line 16 on page 3. If you are not claiming electronic copies, skip to line 17 on page 3.

16. Electronic Copy Circulation		Average No. Copies Each Issue During Preceding 12 Months	No. Copies of Single Issue Published Nearest to Filing Date
a. Paid Electronic Copies	▶	0	0
b. Total Paid Print Copies (Line 15c) + Paid Electronic Copies (Line 16a)	▶	348	404
c. Total Print Distribution (Line 15f) + Paid Electronic Copies (Line 16a)	▶	367	452
d. Percent Paid (Both Print & Electronic Copies) (16b divided by 16c × 100)	▶	95%	89%

☒ I certify that 50% of all my distributed copies (electronic and print) are paid above a nominal price.

17. Publication of Statement of Ownership
☒ If the publication is a general publication, publication of this statement is required. Will be printed in the DECEMBER 2016 issue of this publication. ☐ Publication not required.

18. Signature and Title of Editor, Publisher, Business Manager, or Owner	Date
STEPHEN R. BUSHING - INVENTORY DISTRIBUTION CONTROL MANAGER	9/18/2016

I certify that all information furnished on this form is true and complete. I understand that anyone who furnishes false or misleading information on this form or who omits material or information requested on the form may be subject to criminal sanctions (including fines and imprisonment) and/or civil sanctions (including civil penalties).

PS Form **3526**, July 2014 (Page 3 of 4)

PRIVACY NOTICE: See our privacy policy on www.usps.com

PS Form 3526, July 2014 (Page 1 of 4 (see instructions page 4)) PSN: 7530-01-000-9931   PRIVACY NOTICE: See our privacy policy on www.usps.com

Moving?

Make sure your subscription moves with you!

To notify us of your new address, find your **Clinics Account Number** (located on your mailing label above your name), and contact customer service at:

Email: journalscustomerservice-usa@elsevier.com

800-654-2452 (subscribers in the U.S. & Canada)
314-447-8871 (subscribers outside of the U.S. & Canada)

Fax number: 314-447-8029

Elsevier Health Sciences Division
Subscription Customer Service
3251 Riverport Lane
Maryland Heights, MO 63043

*To ensure uninterrupted delivery of your subscription, please notify us at least 4 weeks in advance of move.

Printed and bound by CPI Group (UK) Ltd, Croydon, CR0 4YY

08/05/2025

01864696-0001